Study Guide
for
Nietzel · Speltz · McCauley · Bernstein

Abnormal Psychology

Prepared by
John Foust
Parkland College

Allyn and Bacon
Boston · London · Toronto · Sydney · Tokyo · Singapore

I am most grateful to my wife, Lynne. It would have been impossible to complete this guide if not for her skill, knowledge dedication, humor, sacrifice, fellowship, and support.

Table of Contents

Preface

Welcome to Abnormal Psychology! If you are like most students, you are probably approaching this course with a mixture of excitement, a strong desire to do well and maybe a bit of apprehension. It is also a safe bet that you have already taken at least one psychology course. If so, you probably already understand that learning occurs most efficiently and effectively when it involves active participation on the part of the learner. Information doesn't simply fly out of a book and into a student's head as he or she reads. If the material is to be understood, absorbed and retained, an active dialogue between student and subject matter is necessary. That is the reason this study guide was written. It has been specifically designed to help you get the most from your textbook and this class, by providing a format for active student participation and, therefore, enhanced understanding.

Your study guide offers activities and suggestions for you to follow before, during and after you have read and studied each chapter.

- **Before you read** a chapter for the first time, you should survey the text to develop a general idea of the topics you will encounter. The *Survey the chapter* section of your study guide will aid you in this process by providing you with a brief overview of each chapter. Read this first and then browse through the chapter to get a feel for the material.

- **As you read** a chapter in the textbook for the first time, it is important for you to actively participate by asking questions and looking for answers. The *Ask questions* section of your study guide will aid you in this process by listing a number of questions which are correlated to the major ideas discussed in the text. You might want to keep these questions handy and as you read your textbook, look for answers.

- **After you read** the chapter, it is time to carefully review and explore the material in detail. Your study guide will aid this process in the *Review and explore the chapter* sections by providing you with a number of short answer, fill-in and matching questions. Use your text to answer these questions. Remember, the more effort you put into it, the better you will understand the material and the more you'll remember later. After you have worked through a section in the study guide and text, use the multiple choice questions in the *Test your understanding* sections to assess your comprehension and reinforce your knowledge.

- **When you have finished** answering the study guide questions, you may wish to look for further material. At the end of each study guide chapter is a section entitled, *Explore the Web to find more information*. This section provides a list of sites on the World Wide Web which correspond to topics discussed in the chapter. Many of the Web pages listed in this guide contain links to other Web sites and more information.

John Foust
Parkland College

CHAPTER 1
Abnormal Behavior: Past and Present Perspectives

Before you read . . .

Survey the chapter

Chapter 1 begins with an entry from the diary of Nelson McGrath. As you read the entry, it quickly becomes obvious that Nelson's thinking is disturbed and his behavior is quite strange and bizarre. The authors of your text then ask a series of questions which form the basis for the rest of this chapter; how should we respond to a person like Nelson McGrath? Should we fear him, condemn him, pity him or envy his imagination? Do we explain his actions by assuming that he is evil? Sick? Inspired?

The remainder of the chapter explores these issues by presenting information on how abnormality has been defined and how people, in various cultures, have reacted to it throughout history. An overview of the major models in use today is presented, including the biological, psychological and sociocultural perspectives.

As you read . . .

Ask questions

1-1   What is abnormal behavior and how has it been defined throughout history?

1-2   How do we view abnormality today?

1-3   What is the biological model and how can it be used to understand abnormal behavior?

1-4   What are the basic structures and functions of the nervous system, brain and neurotransmitters?

1-5   How do genes influence behavior and what research methods are used in behavior genetics?

1-6   What is the psychoanalytical model and how can it be used to understand and treat abnormal behavior?

1-7   What is the behavioral model (learning theory) and how can it be used to understand and treat abnormal behavior?

1-8   What are the cognitive and social-learning models and how can they be used to understand and treat abnormal behavior?

1-9   What is the phenomenological-experimental (humanistic) model and how can it be used to understand behavior?

1-10   What is interpersonal theory and how can it be used to understand and treat abnormal behavior?

1-11   What is the sociocultural model and how can it be used to understand the social and cultural differences in abnormality?

1-12   What is the diathesis-stress model and how can it be used to understand and treat abnormal behavior?

After you read . . .

Review and explore the chapter

| 1-1 | What is abnormal behavior and how has it been defined throughout history? |

1.   How do your authors define abnormal behavior?

2.   Fill in the following.

TIME PERIOD / CULTURE	HOW DID THEY EXPLAIN ABNORMAL BEHAVIOR?	HOW DID THEY RESPOND TO ABNORMAL BEHAVIOR?
Prehistoric times		
Ancient Chinese, Egyptian and Hebrew cultures		
Greek culture		

Roman culture		
Chinese culture (Taoism)		

3.   Match the following.

1.   _b_ Early Middle Ages
2.   _a_ Late Middle Ages
3.   _g_ Avicenna
4.   _e_ Renaissance
5.   _f_ the Age of Enlightenment
6.   _c_ Phillipe Pinel
7.   _h_ Dorothea Dix
8.   _d_ psychoanalysis

a.   witch hunts

b.   period of political and economic upheaval after the fall of the Roman Empire
     (Rationalism and empiricism were replaced by faith that God would reveal divine truths.)

c.   moral treatment

d.   first modern psychological treatment

e.   rise of humanism, confinement in oppressive hospitals and asylums

f.   rapid development of empirical research and science

g.   Islamic physician whose writings helped preserve Greek and Roman learning during the
     Early Middle Ages

h.   mental hygiene movement

1-2	How do we view abnormality today?

4.   Models of abnormality are comprehensive accounts of how and why abnormal behaviors
     _____ (develop / are described) and how best to _____ (treat / avoid) them.

5.   What is the difference between a theory and an hypothesis?

6.   a.   What is a correlational study?

 b.   What does it mean when two variables are positively correlated? Can you think of an example
       of two positively correlated variables?

 c.   What does it mean when two variables are negatively correlated? Can you think of an example
       of two negatively correlated variables?

7.   If you wanted to establish that one variable caused a change in a second variable, would you use a
      correlational study or an experiment? Why?

8.   Match the following.

 1. a d   experiment
 2. d   independent variable
 3. h   dependent variable
 4. e   experimental group
 5. f   confounding variables
 6. g   placebo control
 7. c   quasi-experiment
 8. b   control group

       a.   a research technique where the researcher manipulates one variable and measures the effect
             on a second variable

       b.   group not subjected to the independent variable

       c.   lacks one or more elements of a true experiment

       d.   the variable manipulated by the researcher

       e.   group subjected to the independent variable

       f.   variables that confuse or distort results

g.   additional control group who receive inert treatment

h.   the variable that is observed for change due to the independent variable

---

1-3	What is the biological model and how can it be used to understand abnormal behavior?

9.   What is the basic assumption of the biological model?

10.   The medical model of abnormal behavior considers disturbed behavior to involve _____ (symptoms / a lack) of some underlying illness that is the result of specific causal or _____ (comorbid / etiological) factors.

1-4	What are the basic structures and functions of the nervous system, brain and neurotransmitters?

11.   Match the following.

1.   _b_ central nervous system (CNS)
2.   _e_ peripheral nervous system
3.   _f_ somatic nervous system (SNS)
4.   _c_ autonomic nervous system (ANS)
5.   _a_ sympathetic system
6.   _d_ parasympathetic system

a.   a subsystem of the ANS, it increases physiological arousal

b.   the brain and spinal cord

c.   regulates motivational, emotional and other physical functions

d.   a subsystem of the ANS, it decreases physiological arousal

e.   includes the somatic nervous system and autonomic nervous system

f.   voluntary control of muscles

12.   Fill in the missing function for each of the following brain structures.

BRAIN AREA	BRAIN STRUCTURE	FUNCTION
Hindbrain	medulla	
	reticular formation	
	cerebellum	
Midbrain		
Forebrain	thalamus	
	hypothalamus	
	limbic system	
Cerebrum	cerebral cortex	

13.   a.   What are neurotransmitters?

b.   What is the function of neurotransmitters?

c.   What is the relationship between neurotransmitters and medications used to treat mental disorders?

| 1-5 | How do genes influence behavior and what research methods are used in behavior genetics? |

14. Genes are composed of _____ (alleles (nucleotides)) and are located on the _____ (chromosomes / neurotransmitters). They affect an organism's characteristics indirectly determining the production of _____ (DNA (proteins)). A person's genetic makeup is called the _____ (genotype / phenotype). A person's physical makeup is called the _____ (genotype / phenotype).

15. How are the following research methods used to study genetic influences on behavior?

    a. family studies

    b. adoption studies

    c. twin studies

16. a. Can research on behavior genetics prove whether any particular individual's behavior is due to genes or environment?

    b. Can research on behavior genetics explain the differences between groups of people?

    c. Can research on behavior genetics estimate the average influence that genes and environment exert on individual differences within a group of people?

1-6	What is the psychoanalytical model and how can it be used to understand and treat abnormal behavior?

17.   Match the following.

1.   _c_ psychoanalysis
2.   _a_ id
3.   _d_ ego
4.   _b_ superego

    a.   This structure, which is present at birth, provides the energy (libido) that motivates us. It operates on the pleasure principle.

    b.   This structure is the repository of cultural rules, models of ideal behavior and moral values.

    c.   This psychological model argues that behavior is influenced by unconscious forces. It was developed by Sigmund Freud.

    d.   The personality structure which develops as a child learns that there are limits to id-motivated behavior. It operates on the reality principle.

18.   In your own words, briefly describe each of Freud's psychosexual stages of development.

    a.   oral stage

    b.   anal stage

    c.   phallic stage

    d.   latency period

    e.   genital stage

19.   a.   What is the primary goal of Freudian psychoanalysis?

      b.   List and briefly describe three techniques used in Freudian psychoanalysis.

           1.

           2.

           3.

Test your understanding

1.   Which one of the following statements about abnormal behavior is true?
     a.   All societies agree on what constitutes abnormal behavior.
     b.   The definition of abnormal behavior varies considerably from one society to the next.
     c.   In most cultures the usual way to deal with mental deviates is to lock them up or kill them.
     d.   In most cultures, there is no such thing as abnormal behavior.

2.   In prehistoric and ancient times, abnormal behavior was thought to be caused by
     a.   humors.
     b.   biological factors.
     c.   supernatural forces.
     d.   stress.

3.   Which of the following are incorrectly paired together?
     a.   Early Middle Ages - moral treatment
     b.   Late Middle Ages - witch hunts
     c.   the Age of Enlightenment - rise of empirical research and science
     d.   psychoanalysis - first modern psychological treatment

4.   Which of the following statements about correlational studies is false?
     a.   The longer a person studies, the higher their test score will be. This is an example of a positive correlation.
     b.   Persons with the lowest income have the highest incidence of health problems. This is an example of a negative correlation.
     c.   Correlational studies provide strong evidence of the causal relationships between variables.
     d.   Correlational studies are of little value in the study of abnormal behavior.

5. In an experiment, the group of subjects who are exposed to the independent variable is called the
    a. research group.
    b. independent group.
    c. control group.
    d. experimental group.

6. If you emphasize the fact that all thought and behavior is the result of neural functioning and believe that abnormal behavior is the result of changes in functioning, you are a proponent of the
    a. psychoanalytic model.
    b. biological model.
    c. medical model.
    d. humanistic model.

7. The subsystem of the autonomic nervous system which increases physiological arousal is called the
    a. central nervous system.
    b. somatic nervous system.
    c. sympathetic nervous system.
    d. parasympathetic nervous system.

8. If you sit down to work with this study guide after damaging your cerebellum, you would most likely have a lot of problems
    a. seeing the questions clearly.
    b. understanding the questions you are reading.
    c. remembering the answers.
    d. writing your answers clearly.

9. Higher level cognitive processes take place in the
    a. reticular formation of the brain.
    b. limbic system of the brain.
    c. hypothalamus of the brain.
    d. cerebral cortex of the brain.

10. Which two statements about neurotransmitters are correct?
    a. Neurotransmitters are chemical messengers which cross the synapse between neurons.

    b. Neurotransmitters always stimulate the firing of the neurons they reach.
    c. Neurotransmitters may either stimulate or inhibit the firing of the neurons they reach.
    d. Neurotransmitters may play a role in the production of normal behavior, but they have nothing to do with abnormal behavior.

11. Looking at a photograph of yourself provides information about your
    a. genotype.
    b. phenotype.
    c. DNA.
    d. protein configuration.

12. Research on behavioral genetics
    a. can prove whether any particular individual's behavior is due to genes or environment.
    b. can explain the differences between groups of people.
    c. can estimate the average influence that genes and environment exert on individual differences within a group of people.
    d. is of no value in the study of abnormal behavior.

13. According to the Freudian psychoanalytic model, the _____ ,which is present at birth, operates on the pleasure principle.
    a. id
    b. ego
    c. superego
    d. phallic stage

14. According to the Freudian psychoanalytic model, the _____ is the repository of cultural rules, models of ideal behavior and moral values.
    a. id
    b. ego
    c. superego
    d. oral stage

15. Which of the following is not a technique commonly used in psychoanalytic therapy?
    - a.   rational-emotive therapy
    - b.   free association
    - c.   interpretation of dreams and other behaviors
    - d.   transference

Answers to test your understanding

1. b.   (1-1)
2. c.   (1-1)
3. a.   (1-1)
4. c.   (1-2)
5. d.   (1-2)
6. b.   (1-3)
7. c.   (1-4)
8. d.   (1-4)
9. d.   (1-4)
10. a. c. (1-4)
11. b.   (1-5)
12. c.   (1-5)
13. a.   (1-6)
14. c.   (1-6)
15. a.   (1-6)

1-7	What is the behavioral model (learning theory) and how can it be used to understand and treat abnormal behavior?

20. a.   In your own words, describe the basic assumption on which behaviorists base their study of behavior.

    b.   Briefly describe the focus of each of the following major behavioral theories.

    1.   operant theorists

    2.   theorists emphasizing classical conditioning

    3.   cognitive-behavioral theorists

21.   Match the following.

    1.   _e_ Edward Thorndike
    2.   _e_ B. F. Skinner
    3.   _c_ positive reinforcement
    4.   _f_ negative reinforcement
    5.   _d_ punishment
    6.   _b_ schedules of reinforcement

    a.   proposed that learning follows a law of effect

    b.   reinforcement sometimes intermittent, but still results in persistent behavior

    c.   the act of strengthening a behavior due to the appearance of something pleasant

    d.   a behavioral consequence which makes an action less likely to occur

    e.   developed ideas about the relationship between operant behavior and its observable antecedents and consequences

    f.   the act of strengthening a behavior due to the disappearance of something unpleasant

22.   If a puff of air is directed toward a person's eye, a reflexive eye blink will occur. In the terminology of classical conditioning, the puff is _____ (an unconditioned / a conditioned) stimulus and the blink is _____ (an unconditioned / a conditioned) response.

    A buzzer is sounded and there is no response. At this point, the buzzer is called _____ (a neutral / an unconditioned) stimulus.

    The puff of air is then preceded by the sound of the buzzer. This pairing is made a number of times, until sounding the buzzer alone causes the eye blink to occur. At this point, the buzzer is _____ (an unconditioned / a conditioned) stimulus and the eye blink is _____ (an unconditioned / a conditioned) response.

23.   In your own words, describe the goals and techniques of behavior therapy.

1-8	What are the cognitive and social-learning models and how can they be used to understand and treat abnormal behavior?

24.   a.   In your own words, describe the basic assumptions of the cognitive and social-learning theories.

b.   In your own words, describe each of the following concepts:

1.   observational learning

2.   expectancies

3.   appraisals

4.   attributions

5.   irrational beliefs

25.   According to social-learning and cognitive theories, psychological problems are caused largely by _____ (chemical imbalances in the brain (irrational or distorted thinking)).

1-9   What is the phenomenological-experimental (humanistic) model and how can it be used to understand and treat abnormal behavior?

---

26.   In your own words, describe the basic assumptions of the phenomenological-experimental (humanistic) model.

27.   Briefly describe the basic ideas of the following theorists:

a.   Carl Roger's Self Theory

b.   Abraham Maslow (Humanistic Psychology)

28.   a.   For Rogers, what is necessary if treatment is to be successful?

b.   For Maslow, maladaptive behavior occurs because of what major factor?

1-10	What is interpersonal theory and how can it be used to understand and treat abnormal behavior?

29.   a.   What interpersonal factors tend to produce healthy relationships and personalities according to Sullivan?

b.   What interpersonal factors tend to produce unhealthy relationships and personalities according to Sullivan?

30.   What is the basic assumption on which the interpersonal approach to treatment is based?

1-11	What is the sociocultural model and how can it be used to understand the social and cultural differences in abnormality?

31.   While other models focus on the _____ (internal / external) factors which affect behavior, the sociocultural model concentrates on _____ (internal / external) forces, such as harmful environments, social policies, powerlessness and cultural traditions.

32.   How do the following concepts attempt to explain the social and cultural differences in abnormality?

a.   social causation theory

b.   social drift theory

c.   theory of social relativism

d.   social labeling theory

1-12   What is the diathesis-stress model and how can it be used to understand and treat abnormal behavior?

---

33.   In your own words, briefly describe the diathesis-stress model.

34.   How do theorists who use the diathesis-stress model to understand behavior approach treatment?

Test your understanding

1.   According to the behavioristic model (learning theory), the major factor influencing behavior is
a.   the brain.
b.   genetics.
c.   experience.
d.   free will.

2.   When a behavior is followed by reinforcement, the probability of that behavior happening again
a.   increases (the behavior gets stronger).
b.   decreases (the behavior gets weaker).
c.   may increase or decrease depending on the type of reinforcement used.
d.   remains the same.

3.   During classical conditioning
  a.   some attractive reward is given whenever the desired response occurs.
  b.   an involuntary response is brought under the control of what was, at first, a neutral stimulus.
  c.   a behavior is brought under the control of an unconditioned stimulus.
  d.   behavior remains unchanged.

4.   Cognitive and social learning models differ from traditional learning theory because of the increased emphasis on
  a.   operant conditioning.
  b.   classical conditioning.
  c.   how people process information about their experiences.
  d.   how normal behavior is learned.

5.   Cognitive and social learning models view abnormal behaviors as stemming from
  a.   problems in brain functioning.
  b.   problems which occur mainly in childhood.
  c.   barriers to personal growth due to problematic relationships with others.
  d.   irrational or distorted thinking patterns as a person interprets his or her experiences.

6.   Learning by watching another person's behavior and its consequences is known as
  a.   expectant learning.
  b.   irrational beliefs.
  c.   attribution learning.
  d.   observational learning.

7.   A person seeking phenomenologically based therapy (Carl Rogers) can expect
  a.   a therapeutic environment where he or she can freely and honestly express his or her feelings.
  b.   medication to restore proper brain function.
  c.   to be informed as to why his or her behavior is problematic and how to change it.

  d.   free association and dream interpretation therapy.

8.   Abraham Maslow is associated with
  a.   humanistic psychology and the concept of self-actualization.
  b.   behavioristic psychology and the concept of classical conditioning.
  c.   psychoanalytic psychology and the concept of the role of the unconscious.
  d.   the interpersonal perspective and the importance of how we maintain relationships as we interact with others.

9.   Which of the following best describes the focus of the interpersonal perspective (Sullivan)?
  a.   conditioning
  b.   medication
  c.   relationships
  d.   growth

10. Interpersonal theory seems especially well suited to describe which category of psychological disorders?
  a.   anxiety disorders
  b.   personality disorders
  c.   mood disorders
  d.   disorders of childhood

11. The belief that cultural hardships such as poverty, racism, inferior education, unemployment and social changes put people at a greater risk for behavioral disorders, best describes
  a.   the social causation theory.
  b.   the social drift theory.
  c.   the theory of social relativism.
  d.   social labeling theory.

12. The belief that higher rates of some disorders at lower socioeconomic levels is due to the fact that those lower socioeconomic levels contain a disproportionately high number of persons

with behavior problems is consistent with
a. the social causation theory.
b. the social drift theory.
c. the theory of social relativism.
d. social labeling theory.

13. The belief that standards and definitions of abnormal behavior vary widely in different places and for different groups best describes
a. the social causation theory.
b. the social drift theory.
c. the theory of social relativism.
d. social labeling theory.

14. The basic assumption of the diathesis-stress model is that a behavior disorder results from the combined effects of
a. operant and classical conditioning.
b. conditions of worth and incongruence.
c. predisposition and a stressor.
d. self-actualization and growth needs.

15. According to the diathesis-stress model, the interaction between an individual's characteristics and the environment
a. is ever-changing and dynamic.
b. is constant and unchanging.
c. always produces normal behavior patterns.
d. always produces abnormal behavior patterns.

Answers to test your understanding

1. c.   (1-7)
2. a.   (1-7)
3. b.   (1-7)
4. c.   (1-8)
5. d.   (1-8)
6. d.   (1-8)
7. a.   (1-9)
8. a.   (1-9)
9. c.   (1-10)
10. b.   (1-10)
11. a.   (1-11)
12. b.   (1-11)
13. c.   (1-12)
14. c.   (1-12)
15. a.   (1-12)

When you have finished . . .

Explore the Web to find more information

A general perspective of mental disorders today can be found in **Mental Illness in America, The National Institutes of Mental Health Agenda**. (http://www.nimh.nih.gov/research/amer.htm)

Oregon Health Sciences University and the **National Library of Medicine** maintain **CliniWeb**, a comprehensive Web site. If you go to (http://www.ohsu.edu/cliniweb/A8/A8.html) you will find their **Nervous System** Web page which lists a large number of links to other sites dealing with the brain and nervous system.

If you want in depth information about genetics, go to (**http://www.gdb.org/Dan/DOE/intro.html**).
You will find a **United States Department of Energy** article, " Primer on Molecular Genetics."

A few links to organizations which will provide you with further information and examples of some of the
psychological models that you read about in this chapter are:

- PSYCHODYNAMIC: **FreudNet, The Abraham A. Brill Library** of the New York Psychoanalytic
  Institute (**http://plaza.interport.net/nypsan/**)

- COGNITIVE-BEHAVIORAL: **Behavioral Associates**
  (**http://pages.nyu.edu/~lqh6007/BehavioralAssociates/index.html**)

- COGNITIVE: **Albert Ellis Institute** (**http://www.IRET.org/**)

CHAPTER 2
Assessment and Diagnosis

Before you read . . .

Survey the chapter

Chapter 2 begins with the case of Bill, a 58-year-old business executive, who contacts a clinician because of his concerns. Although he has been financially successful, Bill reports that he is unhappy and anxious. He is concerned about his physical health, his marriage and his job. He worries about the future to the point that he feels depressed and desperate.

The chapter then goes on to discuss questions which are basic to the understanding and treatment of behavioral problems. For example, what constitutes mental disorder? Do Bill's complaints signify the presence of a mental disorder or simply common problems that have gotten out of hand? At first, it may seen that answering questions such as these would be a simple task. As you read this chapter however, you will better understand the complex and often frustrating process of conceptualizing and describing mental disorder.

Information is presented which describes how clinicians, such as Bill's, use various techniques to assess and classify mental disorders. Also discussed, is the frequency with which various mental disorders are diagnosed and how diagnosis is affected by such things as financial and cultural differences.

As you read . . .

Ask questions

2-1   What is a mental disorder? What are the different ways of defining mental disorder?

2-2   What is assessment and diagnosis and what issues influence the quality of assessment and diagnosis?

2-3   How are life records used in assessment?

2-4   How are interviews used in assessment?

2-5   How are psychological tests used in assessment?

2-6   How are observational techniques used in assessment?

2-7   How are biological measures used in assessment?

2-8   What is the DSM classification system and how has it evolved over time?

2-9   What is the DSM-IV and how is it used in diagnosing and classifying behavioral disorders?

2-10   How do real world factors such as socioeconomic or cultural diversity affect the assessment and diagnosis of behavioral disorders?

2-11   How many people currently suffer from a mental disorder or have suffered from one at some point in their lives?

After you read . . .

Review and explore the chapter

2-1   What is a mental disorder? What are the different ways of defining mental disorder?

1.   Why is it difficult to develop a simple and universally useable definition of what constitutes abnormal behavior?

2.   a.   In your own words, describe what is meant when mental disorder is defined as, "a deviation from social expectations."

     b.   Typically, behaviors defined as disorders by this definition are usually quite _____ (common / rare) and are seen by people as _____ (positive / negative).

     c.   What are three problems with this definition?

          1.

          2.

3.

3.   a.   In your own words, describe what is meant when mental disorder is defined as, "what clinicians treat."

b.   The above definition is occasionally used in epidemiology.   What is epidemiology?

c.   What is the greatest strength of this definition?

d.   What are two problems with this definition?

1.

2.

4.   a.   In your own words, describe what is meant when mental disorder is defined as, "the presence of distress or unhappiness."

b.   What are three problems with this definition?

1.

2.

3.

5.   a.   In your own words, describe what is meant when mental disorder is defined as, "a dysfunction which causes harm."

b.   A woman suffering from Alzheimer's disease is often confused because of problems with her memory. Is this an example of a dysfunction or harm? Why?

c.   The person suffering from Alzheimer's disease wanders away from home on a cold day and becomes lost because she can't remember how to get home. Is this an example of a dysfunction or harm? Why?

d.   What are three problems with this definition?

1.

2.

3.

e.   Is this definition useful? Why?

2-2	What is assessment and diagnosis and what issues influence the quality of assessment and diagnosis?

6. a.   _____ (Diagnosing / Assessment) is the process of collecting information for the purpose of making an informed decision. This is often done in order to classify or _____ (diagnose / assess) the nature of a problem.

    b.   What are the three steps which clinicians generally follow in the assessment process?

       1.

       2.

       3.

7. Match the following.

    1.   _c_ reliability
    2.   _b_ test-retest reliability
    3.   _d_ internal consistency
    4.   _a_ interrater reliability

    a.   different clinicians give same diagnosis

    b.   repeated at different times with the same results

    c.   general term describing consistency or agreement among assessment data

    d.   one portion of test is similar to information from other portions of test

8. Match the following.

    1.   _c_ validity
    2.   _a_ content validity
    3.   _d_ predictive validity
    4.   _b_ concurrent validity
    5.   _e_ construct validity

a.   This describes the extent to which a tool measures all aspects that it is supposed to measure.

b.   Two assessment tools, which are given at about the same time, agree.

c.   This general term describes the degree to which an assessment instrument measures what it is supposed to measure.

d.   This describes the ability to correctly forecast behavior.

e.   The results of the assessment instrument agree with what a theory would predict.

9.   Match the following.

1.   _a_ diagnostic sensitivity
2.   _b_ diagnostic specificity
3.   _d_ true positive
4.   _f_ true negative
5.   _e_ false positive
6.   _c_ false negative

a.   The quality of a diagnosis depends on the probability that a person with a mental disorder will be diagnosed as having a disorder.

b.   The quality of a diagnosis depends on the probability that a person without a mental disorder will be diagnosed as having no disorder.

c.   This occurs when a person who is actually suffering from a mental disorder is diagnosed as having no disorder.

d.   This occurs when a person who is actually suffering from a mental disorder is diagnosed as having a disorder.

e.   This occurs when a person who is not suffering from a mental disorder is diagnosed as having a disorder.

f.   This occurs when a person who is not suffering from a mental disorder is diagnosed as having no disorder.

2-3	How are life records used in assessment?

10. a.   What are life records?

b.   Are life records likely to be distorted by a person's attempts to create a special impression?

2-4   How are interviews used in assessment?

---

11. Match the following.

1.   __b__ interview
2.   __a__ structured interview
3.   __c__ mental status examination
4.   __d__ social history

a.   the interviewer asks questions in a predetermined sequence

b.   the most widely used assessment tool for classifying mental disorders

c.   a brief specialized interview designed to assess a person's memory, mood, thinking, etc.

d.   educational achievements, occupational positions, family history, marital status etc.

12. Many clinicians see _____ (structured / unstructured) interviews as too cumbersome and time consuming to use. Structured interviews, however, are believed to be _____ (superior / inferior) to any other tool of diagnostic assessment. Unstructured interviews are almost always _____ (less / more) reliable than structured ones.

2-5   How are psychological tests used in assessment?

---

13. Match the following.

1.   __d__ psychological tests
2.   __f__ norm
3.   __c__ aptitude tests
4.   __b__ achievement tests
5.   __a__ attitude and interest tests
6.   __e__ intelligence tests
7.   __g__ neuropsychological tests
8.   __h__ personality tests

a.   measure the range and strength of a person's interests, attitudes, preferences and values

b.   measure how much a person knows or can do in a specific area

c. measure the accumulated effects of educational or training experience and attempt to predict future performance

d. systematic procedure of observing and describing a person's behavior in a standardized situation

e. measure general mental ability or specific cognitive skills

f. scores used in standardized testing which were obtained from a large number of people who have taken the test under similar circumstances

g. measure problems known to relate to brain dysfunction

h. measure personality traits

14. What is the Minnesota Multiphasic Personality Inventory (MMPI)?

2-6   How are observational techniques used in assessment?

15. Match the following.

1. __b__ observational assessment techniques
2. __d__ naturalistic observation
3. __c__ controlled observation
4. __e__ participant observation
5. __f__ nonparticipant observation
6. __a__ self-monitoring observation

a. client records their own behaviors

b. general term describing an assessment technique popular among behavioral or learning theorists

c. person is observed as they react to a standardized event under the clinician's control

d. observing the person's spontaneous behavior in their everyday environment

e. observer interacts with the client

f. observer does not interact in any way with the client

| 2-7 | How are biological measures used in assessment? |

16. a. What kinds of information can be measured through biological assessment techniques which would be impossible to obtain from other types of measurement techniques?

b. Would you use a CAT scan if you wanted to see the metabolic functioning of the brain? Why or why not? If not, what would you use?

Test your understanding

1. Because there are so many different theoretical perspectives that need to be taken into account when defining mental disorder,
    a. it is difficult to develop a universally useable definition.
    b. it is totally impossible to develop any workable definition.
    c. it is easy to develop a universally useable definition.
    d. there are no useable definitions.

2. Jose is talking loudly to himself in the grocery store. Which definition of mental disorder best applies to Jose's situation?
    a. disorder as a deviation of social expectations
    b. disorder as what clinicians treat
    c. disorder as distress and unhappiness
    d. disorder as dysfunction which causes harm

3. Pat is so afraid that she may have a panic attack at the office that she calls in sick and misses an important meeting. Which of the following definitions of mental disorder best applies to Pat's situation?
    a. mental disorder as a label
    b. mental disorder as what clinicians treat
    c. mental disorder as the presence of distress and unhappiness

d. mental disorder as dysfunction which causes harm

4. A person uses a yardstick to measure a table on Monday and finds that it is exactly 23 inches wide. On Tuesday the same person using the same yardstick measures the table and again it is found to be 23 inches wide. The yardstick has
    a. low reliability.
    b. high test-retest reliability.
    c. high interrater reliability.
    d. high internal reliability.

5. The general term which describes the degree to which an assessment instrument measures what it is supposed to measure is called
    a. diagnostic sensitivity.
    b. reliability.
    c. validity.
    d. diagnostic specificity.

6. A clinician mistakenly diagnoses a patient as having a particular mental disorder, when in actuality the patient has no disorder. This is termed a
    a. true positive.
    b. true negative.
    c. false positive.
    d. false negative.

7. Life records are often useful in assessment, especially when used with other assessment techniques, because
   a. they are higher in validity than most other techniques.
   b. they are less likely to be distorted by a person's attempts to create a special impression.
   c. they are more likely to be distorted by a person's attempts to create a special impression.
   d. they are quicker and easier to use than most other assessment techniques.

8. The most widely used assessment tool for classifying mental disorders
   a. is an interview.
   b. is a brain imagery.
   c. is the MMPI.
   d. is a controlled observation.

9. Structured interviews
   a. are less reliable than unstructured interviews.
   b. are quicker and easier to use than unstructured interviews.
   c. are much more commonly used than are unstructured interviews.
   d. are probably superior not only to unstructured interviews, but to any other diagnostic tool.

10. Which psychological test would best measure how much a person knows or can do in a specific area?
   a. an achievement test
   b. an intelligence test
   c. an aptitude test
   d. a personality test

11. What type of psychological test would best measure the range of a person's interests, attitudes, references and values?
   a. an achievement test
   b. an intelligence test
   c. an aptitude test
   d. a personality test

12. What type of psychological test would best measure general mental or specific cognitive skills?
   a. an achievement test
   b. an intelligence test
   c. an aptitude test
   d. a personality test

13. Observational assessment techniques are especially popular among
   a. psychoanalytic theorists.
   b. neurologically based theorists.
   c. behavioral/learning theorists.
   d. clinicians working with drug abusers.

14. In a participant observation assessment,
   a. the observer interacts with the client.
   b. the observer does not interact in any way with the client.
   c. the client records his or her own behaviors.
   d. the client is not aware of the existence of the observer.

15. Brain imagery techniques such as the CAT, PET or MRI
   a. provide only physical information, so they are of no value in the diagnosis and treatment of mental disorders.
   b. are heavily influenced by the client's self-reports.
   c. are usually low in both reliability and validity.
   d. can provide information about changes in neurological structure and function.

Answers to test your understanding

1.	a.	(2-1)
2.	a.	(2-1)
3.	d.	(2-1)
4.	b.	(2-2)
5.	c.	(2-2)
6.	c.	(2-2)
7.	b.	(2-3)
8.	a.	(2-4)
9.	d.	(2-4)
10.	a.	(2-5)
11.	c.	(2-5)
12.	b.	(2-5)
13.	c.	(2-6)
14.	a.	(2-6)
15.	d.	(2-7)

2-8	What is the DSM classification system and how has it evolved over time?

17. a.   What does the abbreviation DSM stand for?

b.   Who publishes the DSM?

c.   Why was this classification system needed when it was first developed in the 1950's?

18. a.   What major changes were made to the DSM-III and the DSM-III-R in order to correct problems with earlier versions of the DSM?

b.   Even with the above improvements, what were the main weaknesses of the DSM-III and the DSM-III-R?

2-9	What is the DSM-IV and how is it used in diagnosing and classifying behavioral disorders?

19. What method was used in the development of the DSM-IV that was not used in the development of earlier versions of the DSM?

20. Fill in the missing information.

DSM-IV AXIS	ATTRIBUTES DESCRIBED ON THAT AXIS
Axis I	
Axis II	
Axis III	
Axis IV	
Axis V	

21. Match the following.

1. __b__ Disorders Usually First Diagnosed in Infancy, Childhood or Adolescence
2. __c__ Delirium, Dementia, Amnestic and Other Cognitive Disorders
3. __a__ Mental Disorders Due to a General Medical Condition Not Classified Elsewhere
4. __e__ Substance Related Disorders
5. __d__ Schizophrenia and Other Psychotic Disorders

   a.   mental disorders which seem to have a medical condition as their cause

   b.   behavioral problems usually associated with childhood such as learning disorders or attention problems

   c.   impairment of cognitive functioning, often as a result of substance abuse or age

   d.   serious distortions in perception or thinking

   e.   mental disorders arising from dependence on or abuse of drugs

22. Match the following.

1. __b__ Mood Disorders
2. __a__ Anxiety Disorders
3. __d__ Somatoform Disorders

4. __c__ Factitious Disorders
5. __e__ Dissociative Disorders

    a.   "irrational" fear, anxiety, panic and avoidance

    b.   disturbance in emotion (depression and/or mania)

    c.   intentionally creating symptoms of physical or psychological disorder

    d.   physical complaints or symptoms caused by psychological factors

    e.   psychologically caused alteration in identity, consciousness or memory

23. Match the following.

1. __e__ Sexual and Gender Identity Disorders
2. __d__ Eating Disorders
3. __c__ Sleep Disorders
4. __b__ Impulse Control Disorders
5. __a__ Adjustment Disorders
6. __f__ Other Conditions That May Be the Focus of Clinical Attention

    a.   brief periods of poor adaptation to stress

    b.   inability to resist impulse to steal, gamble, set fires, etc.

    c.   insomnia, excessive sleepiness, nightmares or night terrors

    d.   self-starvation or binging and purging of food

    e.   sexual dysfunction or discomfort with one's gender

    f.   conditions which do not fit the criteria for other mental disorders, but are nevertheless problematic

24. Is it possible for a person to meet the criteria for two or more disorders at the same time? Why? What is this called?

25. In your own words, briefly describe what is meant by each of the following criticisms of using the DSM as the basis for diagnosis.

    a.   Labeling produces stereotypes, prejudice and harm.

b.   Mental disorders occur on a continuum, not in discrete categories.

c.   The DSM-IV pays too much attention to reliability and not enough to validity.

d.   A DSM diagnosis implies that disorder is a result of causal factors internal to the person rather than external, environmental problems.

2-10   How do real world factors such as socioeconomic or cultural diversity affect the diagnosis of behavioral disorders?

---

26. In your own words, briefly describe how each of the following could possibly influence the diagnostic process.

a.   insurance

b.   the clinician's professional interests

c.   diagnosis given by non-mental health specialists

27. Match the following examples to the proper concept.

1.   ___ race
2.   ___ ethnicity
3.   ___ culture

a.   American Indian

b.   the "rich"

c.   Italian

28. a.   Why is it sometimes argued that psychological tests may, in general, be biased against ethnic minorities?

b.   What are two specific types of bias that can occur?

1..

2.

29. In your own words, describe why it is important for clinicians to understand a patient's cultural background.

| 2-11 | How many people currently suffer from a mental disorder or have suffered from one at some point in their lives? |

---

30. The total number of people who suffer from a disorder in a specific population is called the _____ (prevalence / incidence) of a disorder. The number of people who develop a disorder in a specific time period (usually the previous 6 or 12 months) is known as the _____ (prevalence / incidence) of a disorder.

31. Each of the following statements is false. Correct each statement to make it true.

a.   The lifetime prevalence for a major mental disorder is less than 10 percent.

b.   The lifetime prevalence of mental disorders is very rarely related to demographic or social variables.

c.   The most common disorders are schizophrenia and depression.

d.   Once a person develops a mental disorder, the symptoms are unrelenting and continuous.

e.   The majority of persons with mental disorders are presently in treatment provided by professional mental health clinicians.

f.   It is rare that a person is diagnosed with two or more mental disorders at the same time.

g.   Most symptoms of mental disorder do not occur until middle age.

Test your understanding

1.   DSM-IV stands for
   a.   Diseases and Symptoms Manual of Abnormal Behavior, 4th ed., which is published by the American Psychological Association.
   b.   Diagnostic and Statistical Manual of Mental Disorders, 4th ed., which is published by the American Psychiatric Association.
   c.   disulfide monochloride - type 4, which is a medication used to treat depression.
   d.   The Department of State Manual no. 4, which laid out the first plans for the classification of mental disorders.

2.   Which two of the following statements about the DSM are totally true?
   a.   The first DSM was developed by the United States military in 1942.
   b.   The edition of the DSM that was first published in 1952 is still in use today.
   c.   The DSM has been revised and updated since it was first published in 1952.
   d.   When using the DSM for diagnoses, a person's behavior is compared to a set of clearly specified criteria for each disorder.

3. The DSM was developed because
   a. there were no diagnostic systems in use at the time.
   b. there were many conflicting systems in use at the time.
   c. a system was needed that was completely free of labeling.
   d. a system was needed that would increase labeling.

4. The DSM-IV differs from earlier versions of the DSM because it was developed using
   a. research based on field trials.
   b. the psychoanalytic approach to describe the cause of mental disorder.
   c. a multiaxial classification system.
   d. no classification system.

5. Which axis of the DSM-IV lists general medical conditions that could be relevant to the understanding or treatment of mental disorder?
   a. Axis II
   b. Axis III
   c. Axis IV
   d. Axis V

6. Which axis of the DSM-IV lists personality disorders?
   a. Axis I
   b. Axis II
   c. Axis III
   d. Axis IV

7. Which axis of the DSM-IV contains sixteen general groups of major mental disorders?
   a. Axis I
   b. Axis II
   c. Axis III
   d. Axis IV

8. The DSM-IV Axis I category, Schizophrenia and Other Psychotic Disorders, includes
   a. mental disorders which seem to have a medical condition as their cause.
   b. behavioral problems usually associated with childhood, such as learning disorders or attention problems.
   c. impairment of cognitive functioning, often as a result of substance abuse or age.
   d. serious distortions in perception or thinking.

9. The DSM-IV Axis I category, Somatoform Disorders, includes
   a. "irrational" fear, anxiety, panic and avoidance.
   b. disturbance in emotion (depression and/or mania).
   c. intentionally creating symptoms of physical or psychological disorder.
   d. physical complaints or symptoms caused by psychological factors.

10. The DSM-IV Axis I category, Impulse Control Disorders, includes
    a. brief periods of poor adaptation to stress.
    b. inability to resist the impulse to steal, gamble, set fires, etc.
    c. insomnia or excessive sleepiness.
    d. self-starvation or binging and purging of food.

11. The term "co-morbid" is used to describe
    a. a situation where the symptoms of a disorder remit and then return again.
    b. a situation where both the patient and the clinician have problems with the same mental disorder.
    c. a situation where the same person shows symptoms of more than one mental disorder.
    d. a situation where two or more family members have the same mental disorder.

12. Which of the following is not one of the major criticisms of the DSM-IV?
    a. The DSM causes labeling, which can negatively distort how a person is seen by others as well as by him or herself.

b.   The symptoms of disorders do not always fit in neat packages.

c.   The diagnostic criteria of the DSM are too simple and specific.

d.   The DSM labels imply that disorder is a result of external, environmental problems, rather than internal ones.

13. Why is it sometimes argued that psychological tests may, in general, be biased against ethnic minorities?

a.   Most psychological tests were developed by whites and normed on white populations.

b.   Most psychological tests were developed by whites and normed on non-white populations.

c.   Most psychological tests were never normed on any group.

d.   Most psychological tests are biased against all ethnic groups.

14. The statement, "About 32 percent of persons in the United States will suffer from a major mental disorder at some point in their lifetime," is an example of

a.   incidence.

b.   prevalence.

c.   co-morbidity.

d.   validity.

15. The most common mental disorders are

a.   schizophrenia and depression.

b.   schizophrenia and obsessive-compulsive disorder.

c.   phobias and alcohol abuse.

d.   alcohol abuse and dissociative identity disorder (multiple personality disorder).

Answers to test your understanding

1.   a.   (2-8)
2.   c. d. (2-8)
3.   b.   (2-8)
4.   a.   (2-9)
5.   b.   (2-9)
6.   b.   (2-9)
7.   a.   (2-9)
8.   d.   (2-9)
9.   d.   (2-9)
10. b   (2-9)
11. c.   (2-9)
12. d.   (2-9)
13. a.   (2-10)
14. b.   (2-11)
15. c.   (2-11)

When you have finished . . .

Explore the Web to find more information

The American Psychological Association's home page (http://www.psych.org/index.html) may be of interest to you.

If you go to (http://www.psych.org/clin_res/q_a.html) you will find the APA's **DSM-IV Questions and Answers** page. A few of the topics discussed there which relate to this chapter are:

When did the DSM-IV become official?

Sometimes different disorders or subtypes of disorders have the same diagnostic code. Is there an error here?

How can I quickly find out the changes between the DSM-III-R and the DSM-IV?

I've noticed that the criterion, "the disturbance causes clinically significant distress or impairment in social, occupational, or other important areas of functioning," has been added to the criteria sets for many mental disorders. Why was this done?

I understand that there is a primary care version of the DSM-IV-- please tell me about it.

Whom do I contact if I find a mistake or inconsistency in the DSM-IV?

How do I order copies of the DSM-IV?

The Department of Clinical and Applied Psychology, University of Bonn, Germany maintains a very comprehensive Web site at (**http://www.psychologie.uni-bonn.de/kap/links_20.htm**). To find links to many of the topics discussed in this chapter, click on <u>Assessment</u>.

Internet Mental Health provides an article, "Prevalence of Mental Disorders," The Harvard Medical School Mental Health Letter, April, 1989. You can access this article by going to (**http://www.mentalhealth.com/mag1/p5h-mh02.html**).

CHAPTER 3
Disorders of Infancy, Childhood, and Adolescence

Before you read . . .

Survey the chapter

Chapter 3 deals with behavioral disorders which commonly begin or are diagnosed in childhood. The chapter begins with the case of Tom, a child who is having problems both at school and at home. Tom seems inattentive at school and although he is intelligent, he is doing poorly. He is forgetful, at times anxious and often complains of physical problems. Because of their concerns, Tom's parents contact a clinical psychologist. They are confused. Is Tom's behavior abnormal? Does his behavior signal the onset of other problems? Will he "grow out of it"? Is all of this due to something they are doing or maybe not doing?

This chapter deals with the issues which surround these questions. It begins by discussing general information about child development and psychopathology. The bulk of this chapter discusses specific disorders, including oppositional defiant disorder, conduct disorder, attention-deficit/hyperactivity disorder, mood and anxiety disorders, eating disorders and elimination disorders.

As you read . . .

Ask questions

3-1   How has the study of developmental psychopathology helped in increasing our understanding of behavioral disorders?

3-2   How are children's disorders classified and diagnosed?

3-3   Are disruptive behaviors and attention-deficit/hyperactivity disorder a major problem in the United States today?

3-4   What is oppositional defiant disorder?

3-5   What is conduct disorder?

3-6   What causes conduct disorder?

3-7   How are disruptive disorders such as conduct disorder and oppositional defiant disorder treated?

3-8   What is attention-deficit/hyperactivity disorder (ADHD)?

3-9   In an attempt to better understand the causes of attention-deficit/hyperactivity disorder, what factors are presently under investigation?

3-10   How is attention-deficit/hyperactivity disorder treated?

3-11   What other internalizing disorders occur in childhood or adolescence?

3-12   What is separation anxiety disorder?

3-13   What causes separation anxiety disorder?

3-14   How is separation anxiety disorder treated?

3-15   How does depression typically occur in childhood and adolescence?

3-16   What factors influence the development of childhood depression?

3-17   How is childhood depression treated?

3-18   What are anorexia nervosa and bulimia nervosa?

3-19   What factors influence the development of anorexia nervosa and bulimia nervosa?

3-20   How are anorexia nervosa and bulimia nervosa treated?

3-21   What are elimination disorders and how are they treated?

After you read . . .

Review and explore the chapter

3-1	How has the study of developmental psychopathology helped in increasing our understanding of behavioral disorders?

1.   What two factors have occurred in the last few years which have lead to the development of developmental psychopathology?

a.

b.

2. a. What do developmental psychologists mean by the concept of developmental tasks?

    b. Can you think of examples of developmental tasks?

    c. What is the relationship between how a child deals with developmental tasks at an early age and that child's later development?

3. What is the relationship between developmental tasks and the later development of maladaptive behavior?

4. a. What is "The Strange Situation" assessment?

    b. What relationship patterns indicate secure attachment?

    c. What relationship patterns indicate insecure attachment?

d. _____ (Secure / Insecure) attachment is correlated to an increased risk for behavioral problems in later childhood.

| 3-2 | How are children's disorders classified and diagnosed? |

5. a. In your own words, describe the categorical approach to classifying childhood disorders.

    b. What is an example of this approach?

6. a. In your own words, describe the dimensional approach to classifying childhood disorders.

    b. What is meant by the concept of externalizing problems (CBCL checklist)?

    c. What is meant by the concept of internalizing problems (CBCL checklist)?

| 3-3 | Are disruptive behaviors and attention-deficit/hyperactivity disorder a major problem in the United States today? |

7. Disruptive behaviors and attention deficits are _____ (the most / the least) common reasons for a child's referral to a mental health facility, accounting for _____ (25-35 / 60-70) percent of child and adolescent cases.

8. Disruptive disorders such as oppositional defiant disorder and conduct disorder, as well as some aspects of attention-deficit/hyperactivity disorder would be described on the _____ (externalizing / internalizing) dimension of the Child Behavior Checklist.

| 3-4 | What is oppositional defiant disorder? |

9. List four behaviors which are often seen in oppositional defiant disorder.

    a.

    b.

    c.

    d.

10. How does the DSM-IV differentiate between ODD and common behavioral problems in children?

11. a. Using what has been learned through longitudinal research, what can you predict about further conduct problems in preschoolers and grade schoolers showing oppositional defiant disorder symptoms?

    b. What factors would you look for which would indicate that present disruptive behaviors will continue as the child ages?

| 3-5 | What is conduct disorder? |

12. How does conduct disorder differ from oppositional defiant disorder?

13. Summarize the symptoms of conduct disorder on the table below.

CATEGORY	SUMMARY OF BEHAVIORS
Aggression to people and animals	bullies and threatens others, initiates and uses weapon in fights, cruelty to others and animals, stealing, forcing someone into sexual activity
Destruction of property	
Deceitfulness or theft	
Serious violation of rules	

14. Studies suggest that youngsters who show childhood onset (before age 10) of conduct disorder are _____ (more / less) likely to experience academic failure and develop adult antisocial problems. Later onset conduct disorder is _____ (more / less) likely to dissipate by the end of the teenage years.

3-6	What causes conduct disorder?

15. In your own words, describe how the following biological factors may contribute to the development of conduct disorder?

a.   testosterone levels

b.   neurotransmitters

c.   physiological arousal

16. In your own words, describe how the following cognitive and psychosocial factors may contribute to the development of conduct disorder?

a.   deficits in neurological abilities such as memory, problem solving and language

b.   parenting skills

c.   an adverse environment

d.   a child's social-cognitive skills

3-7   How are disruptive disorders such as conduct disorder and oppositional defiant disorder treated?

17. a.   What is the focus of programs designed to improve specific parenting skills, such as Eyberg's Parent-Child Interaction Therapy?

b.   Does it work?

c.   List three possible problems with the parent training approach.

1.

2.

3.

18. a.   What is the focus of cognitive-behavioral programs which are designed to treat disruptive disorders?

    b.   How effective are cognitive-behavioral approaches in dealing with the long-term progress of conduct disorder?

| 3-8 | What is attention-deficit/hyperactivity disorder (ADHD)? |

19. What are the three core symptoms of attention-deficit/hyperactivity disorder? Give an example of each.

    a.   example:

    b.   example:

    c.   example:

20. How does the DSM-IV differentiate attention-deficit/hyperactivity disorder from common disruptive actions seen from time to time in all children?

21. About _____ (3-5 / 15-20) percent of school-aged children in the United States meet the formal DSM-IV criteria for ADHD. _____ (Boys / Girls)are more often diagnosed and prevalence rates are slightly more common among _____ (lower / higher) socioeconomic classes.

22. Mark the following with ADHD-I if it is more commonly seen in ADHD inattention type and ADHD-H if it is more common in ADHD hyperactivity / impulsivity type.

    a. _____ low popularity among peers

    b. _____ more likely associated with the presence of learning disabilities

    c. _____ four to five times more common than the other type

    d. _____ girls more inclined to show this type

    e. _____ internalizing behavior problems

    f. _____ externalizing behavior problems

23. Billy is in the fourth grade and meets the criteria for ADHD. Based on prevalence rates, what would you predict for Billy by the time he reaches adolescence? Adulthood?

3-9 In an attempt to better understand the causes of attention-deficit/hyperactivity disorder, what factors are presently under investigation?

---

24. How do the following biological factors influence the development of attention-deficit/hyperactivity disorder?

    a. prenatal and birth problems

    b. genetic factors

    c. the reticular activating system of the brain

    d. the frontal lobes

25. What patterns of parent-child interaction may possibly combine with biological predispositions to increase the likelihood of developing ADHD?

3-10   How is attention-deficit/hyperactivity disorder treated?

---

26. a.   Why are stimulant medications commonly used in the treatment of ADHD?

    b.   Do they work well in most cases?

    c.   What problems are associated with the use of stimulant medications?

27. What are two commonly used psychological treatments for ADHD?

Test your understanding

1.   Which two of the following statements about developmental tasks are true?
    a.   Developmental tasks have no relationship to later development.
    b.   Developmental tasks are the basic building blocks upon which a child's later adjustment begins.
    c.   Developmental tasks do not occur in infancy because babies don't understand them.
    d.   Developmental tasks are important from infancy through adolescence.

2.   An infant who is unable to negotiate the developmental task of using the parent as a source of comfort during stressful situations,
    a.   is less likely to become self-reliant as a preschooler.
    b.   is more likely to become self-reliant as a preschooler.
    c.   is suffering from oppositional defiant disorder.
    d.   is suffering from conduct disorder.

3. An example of a categorical approach for classifying childhood psychopathology is
    a. externalizing problems.
    b. internalizing problems.
    c. the DSM-IV.
    d. none of the above.

4. The most common reasons for a child's referral to a mental health facility are
    a. depression and sleep problems.
    b. depression and anxiety.
    c. disruptive behaviors and attention deficits.
    d. issues involving developmental task problems.

5. Which of the following is not typical of oppositional defiant disorder?
    a. very poor control over emotions
    b. noncompliant and argumentative behavior
    c. blaming others for their own mistakes
    d. dependence on others for decision making

6. The behaviors associated with conduct disorder
    a. are potentially harmful to the child, others or property.
    b. are less disruptive than with oppositional defiant disorder.
    c. are easily treated.
    d. rarely impact on the child's ability to function well in the family or at school.

7. Which of the following is not typical of conduct disorder?
    a. intentionally destroying property
    b. running away and truancy
    c. cruelty to others
    d. suicide attempts

8. Which two of the following statements about the causes of conduct disorder are true?
    a. Studies consistently show that genetics play no role in the development of conduct disorder.
    b. Children with conduct disorder often have problems processing and using language.
    c. The development of conduct disorders seems to be unaffected by the mother or father's parenting skills.
    d. Aggressive children tend to have problems thinking of nonaggressive ways of solving problems.

9. Parent-Child Interaction Therapy focuses on
    a. genetic counseling.
    b. coaching parents on how to play and talk effectively with their children.
    c. teaching children how to relate to their parents.
    d. the nonverbal communication between parents and their children.

10. Which of the following is not one of the core symptoms of ADHD?
    a. inattention
    b. hyperactivity
    c. impulsivity
    d. aggression

11. About what percentage of school-aged children in the United States meet the criteria for ADHD?
    a. 3-5 percent
    b. 10-15 percent
    c. 20-25 percent
    d. 40-50 percent

12. ADHD children with hyperactivity
    a. are more likely to be girls.
    b. are more likely to also have sensory-motor problems and learning disorders.
    c. are more likely to also have conduct disorder.
    d. are more likely to have other internalizing problems such as anxiety and depression.

13. As with the disruptive disorders, ADHD seems to be caused
    a. entirely by environmental factors such as family stress and adversity.
    b. entirely by limited cognitive and social skills.
    c. by poor parenting skills.
    d. by a combination of biological, environmental and cognitive factors.

14. Which of the following statements about the use of medications to treat the core symptoms of ADHD is true?
    a. Only about 25 percent of children show positive results with medication.
    b. The most commonly used drugs are depressants.
    c. The most commonly used drugs are stimulants.
    d. The best thing about using medications to treat ADHD is that there are no side effects.

15. Oppositional defiant disorder, conduct disorder and ADHD indicate a risk for continuing antisocial problems especially
    a. if they are treated with medication.
    b. if they are not treated with medication.
    c. if the child shows signs of these disorders at an early age.
    d. if the child shows the first signs of one of these in later childhood or adolescence.

Answers to test your understanding

1. b. d. (3-1)
2. a.   (3-1)
3. c.   (3-2)
4. c.   (3-3)
5. d.   (3-4)
6. a.   (3-5)
7. d.   (3-5)
8. b. d. (3-6)
9. b.   (3-7)
10. d.   (3-8)
11. a.   (3-8)
12. c.   (3-8)
13. d.   (3-9)
14. c.   (3-10)
15. c.   (3-10)

3-11   What other internalizing disorders occur in childhood or adolescence?

---

28. Children suffer anxiety and mood disorders that are very _____ (similar to / different from) those diagnosed in adults.

29. a. Are anxiety disorders common in childhood?

b.   What two criteria must be present in order for anxiety to be severe enough to be diagnosed as symptomatic of a mental disorder?

30. Anxiety consists of what three factors?

a.

b.

c.

| 3-12 | What is separation anxiety disorder? |

31. In the blank areas of the table below, fill in the remaining behaviors which indicate separation anxiety disorder.

	BEHAVIORS ASSOCIATED WITH SEPARATION ANXIETY DISORDER
1.	child is clingy and dependent on adults, demanding help for even the simplest tasks
2.	
3.	
4.	
5.	
6.	
7.	

32. Refusal to go to school can be caused by separation anxiety disorder or social and simple phobia. Differentiate between these two causes.

33. What specific early childhood characteristic often indicates a predisposition for fearfulness and an increased chance to develop separation anxiety disorder?

3-13   What causes separation anxiety disorder?

34. In your own words, describe how the following factors may play a role in the development of separation anxiety disorder?

    a.   biological factors

    b.   environmental factors

    c.   cognitive factors

3-14   How is separation anxiety disorder treated?

35. In your own words, describe how systematic desensitization therapy is used in the treatment of separation anxiety disorder.

36. In your own words, describe how cognitive therapy is used in the treatment of separation anxiety disorder.

37. In your own words, describe how medications are used in the treatment of separation anxiety disorder.

| 3-15 | How does depression typically occur in childhood and adolescence? |

38. Summarize the symptoms of childhood depression on the table below.

SYMPTOM CATEGORY	SPECIFIC BEHAVIORS
Mood / negative feelings	irritability, sadness, hopelessness
Health	
View of self / environment	
Relationships with others	
Self-destructive tendencies	

| 3-16 | What factors influence the development of childhood depression? |

39. In your own words, describe how each of the following relate to the development of childhood depression.

a.   brain activity

b.   genetic factors

c.   affect regulation

| 3-17 | How is childhood depression treated? |

40. a.   What are two reasons why tricyclic antidepressant medications should be given to children only if they have failed to respond to other treatments?

b.   What treatments, other than medication, seem to produce significant improvement in children with mild depression?

3-18   What are anorexia nervosa and bulimia nervosa?

41. Mark the following with AN if it is more commonly seen in anorexia nervosa and BN if it is more common in bulimia nervosa.

a.   _____ amenorrhea

b.   _____ binge eating as an essential feature

c.   _____ distorted body image

d.   _____ persons are often of normal weight or possibly even overweight

e.   _____ motivation is the avoidance of perceived fatness rather than the desire to be extremely thin

---

3-19   What factors influence the development of anorexia nervosa and bulimia nervosa?

42. In your own words, describe how each of the following attempt to explain the development of anorexia nervosa and bulimia nervosa.

a.   sociocultural explanations

b.   psychoanalytic explanations

c.   biological explanations

43. What specific factor, which does not seem to play a significant role in anorexia nervosa, seems to be particularly important in the development of bulimia nervosa?

44. Most preadolescent anorectics have had one or more _____ (internalizing / externalizing) problem behaviors prior to their eating disturbance.

| 3-20 | How are anorexia nervosa and bulimia nervosa treated? |

---

45. In your own words, describe how each of the following are used in the treatment of anorexia nervosa and bulimia nervosa.

   a. medication

   b. behavior therapy

   c. family therapy

| 3-21 | What are elimination disorders and how are they treated? |

---

46. Elimination disorders include _____ (enuresis / encopresis), which is the release of urine into bedding or clothes and _____ (enuresis / encopresis), which is the repeated passage of feces into inappropriate places.

47. Although the causes of enuresis are not clearly understood, it can be effectively treated. What are three methods used to treat enuresis?

   a.

   b.

   c.

48. What are two common methods used in the treatment of encopresis?

Test your understanding

1. Anxiety and mood disorders during childhood and adolescence
    a.   are both examples of internalizing problems.
    b.   are rarely comorbid with each other.
    c.   are very commonly and effectively treated with medications.
    d.   are not effectively treated with cognitive-behavioral techniques.

2. Which of the following is not a factor commonly seen in anxiety?
    a.   observable avoidance behaviors
    b.   physiological arousal
    c.   cognitive arousal (worry)
    d.   encopresis

3. Which of the following statements about separation anxiety disorder is false?
    a.   The child displays excessive fear of being left alone.
    b.   The child rarely reports physical complaints.
    c.   The child commonly suffers from nightmares.
    d.   The child often refuses to go to school.

4. What characteristic in early childhood often indicates a predisposition for fearfulness and an increased chance to develop separation anxiety disorder?
    a.   tolerance
    b.   late speech development
    c.   inhibition
    d.   early onset conduct disorder

5. If someone asked you what causes separation anxiety disorder (SAD), the most accurate answer would be
    a.   that SAD is totally a biologically based problem.
    b.   that SAD is caused by poor parenting skills.
    c.   that SAD is caused by inaccurate perceptions and thoughts on the part of the child.
    d.   that SAD is probably influenced by a combination of biological, environmental and cognitive factors.

6. Having the child apply anxiety reducing techniques, while gradually increasing exposure to threatening separation situations, describes which therapeutic technique?
    a.   desensitization therapy
    b.   cognitive therapy
    c.   parental skills training
    d.   social learning therapy

7. Childhood depression
    a.   is extremely rare.
    b.   affects only mood.
    c.   can affect mood, relationships with friends and how the child views him or herself.
    d.   is not treatable.

8. The rate of depression occurring in children of depressed biological parents is _____ the rate for children in the general population.
    a.   much lower than
    b.   a little lower than
    c.   about the same as
    d.   higher than

9. Which of the following statements about the treatment of childhood depression is false?
    a. Recent studies question the effectiveness of tricyclic antidepressants when treating childhood depression.
    b. Negative side effects are an important concern when using medications such as tricyclic antidepressants to treat childhood depression.
    c. Some of the common cognitive-behavioral treatments used in treating childhood depression include cognitive restructuring and coping skills training.
    d. Cognitive-behavioral treatments are not very effective in the treatment of childhood depression.

10. Distorted body image is common in
    a. childhood depression.
    b. separation anxiety disorder.
    c. anorexia nervosa.
    d. bulimia nervosa.

11. Binge eating is an essential feature of
    a. childhood depression.
    b. separation anxiety disorder.
    c. anorexia nervosa.
    d. bulimia nervosa.

12. Which of the following statements about the causes of eating disorders is false?
    a. Society bombards us with the message that slimness is necessary for beauty and acceptance. This may create unreasonable expectations.
    b. Some researchers believe that eating disorders may be a method of avoiding and diverting attention from family conflicts.
    c. Many researchers believe that learning plays a greater role in the development of anorexia nervosa than it does in the development of bulimia nervosa.
    d. Some researchers point out that brain dysfunction may predispose a person to develop an eating disorder.

13. Which of the following statements about the treatment of eating disorders is true?
    a. By far, the most effective treatment for both anorexia nervosa and bulimia nervosa is antidepressant medications.
    b. By far, the most effective treatment for both anorexia nervosa and bulimia nervosa is systematic desensitization.
    c. By far, the most effective treatment for both anorexia nervosa and bulimia nervosa is family therapy.
    d. Most techniques have met with mixed results. There is no one superior treatment.

14. Encopresis is
    a. the release of urine into bedding or clothes.
    b. the repeated passage of feces into inappropriate places.
    c. a rare form of bulimia nervosa.
    d. a drug used to treat childhood depression.

15. Which of the following is commonly used in the treatment of enuresis?
    a. a urine alarm
    b. a feces alarm
    c. parental skills training
    d. Nothing. Enuresis is not treatable.

Answers to test your understanding

1. a. (3-11)
2. d. (3-11)
3. b. (3-12)
4. c. (3-12)
5. d. (3-13)
6. a. (3-14)
7. c. (3-15)
8. d. (3-16)
9. d. (3-17)

10. c.   (3-18)
11. d.   (3-18)
12. d.   (3-19)
13. d.   (3-20)
14. b.   (3-21)
15. a.   (3-21)

When you have finished . . .

Explore the Web to find more information

A good place to start your search for information on childhood disorders is **The American Academy of Child and Adolescent Psychiatry's** Web site which is located at (**http://www.aacap.org/web/aacap/**). When you arrive, click on <u>Facts for Families</u>, which will take you to a series of over 50 informative fact sheets designed to provide information and help for children and their families.

There is a wealth of information on the net about attention-deficit/hyperactivity disorder. Some of the best links are:

- The **Children and Adults with Attention Deficit Disorders** (CH.A.D.D.) home page. (**http://www.chadd.org/**)

- The **National Institutes of Mental Health's** document, "Attention Deficit Hyperactivity Disorder" (**http://www.nimh.nih.gov/publicat/adhd.htm**) is detailed and especially informative.

- **One A.D.D. Place** (**http://www.greatconnect.com/oneaddplace/**)

If you are looking for more information on Tourette Syndrome, the **National Tourette Syndrome Association, Inc.** site is located at (**http://neuro-www2.mgh.harvard.edu/tsa/tsamain.nclk**).

Another good T.S. site is **The Tourette Syndrome Home Page**. (**http://www-personal.umd.umich.edu/~infinit/tourette.html**)

If you are looking for more information on childhood depression, try the following sites:

- "Depression Rx for Teens No Longer 'Hit or Miss'?," by Pauline Anderson, The Medical Post, February 20, 1996. (**http://www.mentalhealth.com/mag1/p5m-dp02.html**)

- "Can Adolescent Suicide Be Prevented?," The Harvard Medical School Mental Health Letter, November 1989. (**http://www.mentalhealth.com/mag1/p5h-sui4.html**)

- The <u>Facts for Families</u> link on **The American Academy of Child and Adolescent Psychiatry** home page mentioned earlier has a number of articles dealing with childhood depression.

If you are looking for eating disorders information, one of the best places to begin your search is **The Something Fishy Website on Eating Disorders**. (**http://www.something-fishy.com/ed.htm**)

Another good place for information on eating disorders is the **Anorexia Nervosa and Bulimia Association** (ANAB) in Canada. Their URL is (**http://qlink.queensu.ca/~4map/anabhome.htm**).

CHAPTER 4
Developmental and Learning Disabilities

Before you read . . .

Survey the chapter

Chapter 4 deals with problems which can disrupt a child's ability to develop language skills, motor skills, cognitive abilities, or necessary adaptive and social behaviors normally. The effects of these disabilities can be devastating and long lasting. The chapter begins with the case of Jordan, an eleven year old boy with severe mental retardation and cerebral palsy. As you will see, the cluster of problems which affect Jordan's development have far reaching implications for Jordan as well as his family.

Mental retardation is discussed, as well as autism, which you will see is a spectrum disorder which comes in different forms. These disorders are described and various views concerning their etiology and treatment are presented. In the last section, learning disabilities and reading disabilities are described. Their causes and treatment are also covered.

As you read . . .

Ask questions

4-1   What do clinicians mean when they talk about developmental disabilities?

4-2   How is mental retardation defined?

4-3   How is mental retardation classified?

4-4   How can organic factors such as genetic problems influence the development of specific types of mental retardation?

4-5   Can environmental factors cause organic damage which can lead to mental retardation?

4-6   Can psychosocial factors influence the development of mental retardation?

4-7   Can mental retardation be prevented?

4-8   How can mental retardation be treated?

4-9   What is autism?

4-10   What are the features of autism in its typical form?

4-11   What factors influence the development of autism in its typical form?

4-12   What are some of the atypical forms of autism?

4-13   How are pervasive developmental disorders treated?

4-14   How are learning disabilities defined and identified?

4-15   What factors influence the development of reading disabilities?

4-16   How are learning disabilities and reading problems treated?

After you read . . .

Review and explore the chapter

4-1	What do clinicians mean when they talk about developmental disabilities?

1. a. What are the three criteria which must be met according to the legal definition of developmental disability?

    1.

    2.

    3.

    b. Most developmental disabilities are diagnosed in _____ (infancy and early childhood / adolescence and early adulthood).

2.   a.   In your own words, define "domains of development."

b.   How are developmental domains used to measure developmental disabilities?

c.   List the four major developmental domains.

   1.

   2.

   3.

   4.

3.   Match the following.

   1.   ____ gross motor skills
   2.   ____ fine motor skills
   3.   ____ visual-motor skills
   4.   ____ expressive language
   5.   ____ receptive language
   6.   ____ cognition
   7.   ____ habituation speed
   8.   ____ mental age
   9.   ____ adaptive behaviors

   a.   key domain efficiently predicted by family information before age three, after age three intelligence tests often used

b.   domain is often measured through observations of parents or teachers

c.   the understanding of language

d.   the amount of time taken by an infant to lose interest in a stimulus

e.   on intelligence tests, the average number of questions "passed" by persons of a certain age

f.   language used to communicate one's thoughts

g.   hand-eye coordination

h.   control of large bodily movements

i.   control of upper extremity and hand and finger movements

---

4-2   How is mental retardation defined?

4.   How is mental retardation defined in this chapter?

5.   a.   What two issues have long been debated concerning attempts to define mental retardation?

     1.

     2.

b.   In your own words, briefly describe the long lasting problem of using IQ scores to distinguish retarded from normal functioning.

c.   Are IQ scores the only criterion for determining mental retardation today?

4-3	How is mental retardation classified?

6. Identify the following as, mild, moderate, severe or profound mental retardation.

   1. ____ IQ range of approximately 35-40 to 50-55

   2. ____ IQ range of approximately 20-25 to 35-40

   3. ____ IQ range of approximately 50 to 70-75

   4. ____ IQ range below 20-25

   5. ____ slower-than-average developmental rate often overlooked until middle childhood or adolescence; as adults, most marry and live independently

   6. ____ very limited early childhood communication, acquisition of simple speech by middle childhood, by adulthood, may recognize a few words, most do not learn to read; assistance needed for self-care

   7. ____ acquisition of speech is unlikely, many are wheelchair-bound due to gross motor deficits

   8. ____ delays in language acquisition, but most acquire expressive language; as adults, very few marry, commonly live in supervised group homes

4-4	How can organic factors such as genetic problems influence the development of specific types of mental retardation?

7. Organic causes of mental retardation account for _____ (25-50 percent / 50-75 percent) of all retardation cases, most with IQs _____ (above / below) 50.

8. Fill in the missing information.

DOWN SYNDROME	
Description of chromosomal abnormality	
Description of physical characteristics	
Effect of "aging process"	

Description of typical social characteristics	
Common IQ range	
Description of typical level of adaptation	

9.   Fill in the missing information.

FRAGILE X SYNDROME	
Description of chromosomal abnormality	
Description of typical physical characteristics	
Typical social characteristics	
Common IQ range	varies, cognitive effects more severe in males
Description of typical level of adaptation	varies, effects more severe in males

10.   Fill in the missing information.

WILLIAMS SYNDROME	
Description of chromosomal abnormality	
Behavioral limitations	
Description of typical physical characteristics	

11. Fill in the missing information.

PHENYLKETONURIA - PKU	
Effect on protein metabolism due to inherited gene mutation	
Common IQ range if untreated	
Common IQ range if detected early and treated	
Description of typical behavioral characteristics	

4-5   Can environmental factors cause organic damage which can lead to mental retardation?

---

12. a.   What are teratogens?

     b.   In your own words, briefly describe the typical features of fetal alcohol syndrome.

13. What environmental events, other than the effects of teratogens, may cause organic problems which lead to mental retardation?

4-6   Can psychosocial factors influence the development of mental retardation?

---

14. It is believed that adversity in a child's psychosocial environment can limit intellectual development, although the effects are usually confined to the _____ (mild / moderate / severe / profound) range of retardation. The term _____ (environmental deprivation / cultural-familial) is used to describe mild mental retardation without a known organic etiology. Many researchers are focusing on

environmental deprivation conditions where parents _____ (are absent from the home / have limited intellectual skills or little education).

4-7   Can mental retardation be prevented?

15. Briefly describe and give examples for each of the following prevention programs.

a.   genetic counseling

b.   prevention techniques designed to foster good physical and psychological health

c.   early detection

d.   Project Head Start

4-8   How can mental retardation be treated?

16. Interventions for mental retardation are not usually aimed at "cures." Instead, most interventions focus on three goals. Please list these goals.

a.

b.

c.

17. In your own words, briefly describe how behavior modification programs can be used to increase adaptive skills or decrease self-injurious or disruptive behaviors.

18. In your own words, briefly describe how self-instruction can be used to increase adaptive skills.

19. What are two possible reasons why self-injurious behavior is so difficult to eliminate in persons with mental retardation?

    a.

    b.

20. Prior to the 1970's, children in the United States were usually placed in _____ (a group home / an institution) for long-term care. In the 1970's, such beliefs were replaced by faith in the benefits of _____ (normalization / mainstreaming), which was the idea that persons with mental retardation should experience the "norms and patterns of the mainstream society" in their everyday lives. Normalization and deinstitutionalization put increased responsibility on neighborhood schools to educate _____ (all children with mental retardation / those children with mild or moderate retardation). As a response, most children with mental retardation were placed in _____ (special schools / self-contained classrooms in regular public schools). Opposition to this approach has steadily _____ (decreased / increased) in the past two decades, which has consequently led many school districts to initiate a policy of _____ (normalization / mainstreaming), where children with mental retardation are served in regular classrooms if possible.

Test your understanding

1. Which of the following is not one of the three criteria which describe developmental disabilities according to the legal definition?
    a. lifelong impairment in mental or physical functioning that first becomes evident prior to adulthood
    b. substantial limitations in daily living skills such as communication and self-care
    c. IQ score below 70 if under age 10, 75 if older than age 10
    d. necessity for extended specialized care

2. Most developmental disabilities are diagnosed in
    a. infancy and early childhood.
    b. early childhood and adolescence.
    c. adolescence and early adulthood.
    d. adulthood.

3. The concept of receptive language refers to
    a. gestures.
    b. the understanding of language.
    c. language used to communicate one's thoughts.
    d. cognitive "self-talk."

4. The amount of time taken by an infant to lose interest in a stimulation is called
    a. hand-eye coordination.
    b. adaptive behavior lag.
    c. habituation speed.
    d. boredom.

5. What two factors are commonly used today in determining mental retardation?
    a. IQ and mental age
    b. mental age and adaptive functioning
    c. genetic testing and parental surveys
    d. IQ and adaptive functioning

6. Which of the following best describes an IQ in the range of approximately 35 or 40-50, a delay in language acquisition and functioning levels which commonly result in living in group homes as adults?
    a. mild mental retardation
    b. moderate mental retardation
    c. severe mental retardation
    d. profound mental retardation

7. Which of the following best describes an IQ in a range below 20 to 25, the level of retardation where deficits are most dramatic.
    a. mild mental retardation
    b. moderate mental retardation
    c. severe mental retardation
    d. profound mental retardation

8. Down syndrome is caused by
    a. a genetic problem in which the 21st pair of chromosomes fail to separate resulting in three chromosomes (trisomy).
    b. a heritable genetic mutation on the X chromosome.
    c. a missing gene on chromosome 7.
    d. head injury in combination with poor nutrition.

9. Children with fragile X syndrome
    a. have a missing gene on chromosome 7.
    b. suffer from premature aging.
    c. lack interest in social relationships.
    d. typically suffer from greater deficits if they are female.

10. In which type of mental retardation is one more likely to see a child with an elfin-like appearance who has vocabulary and hearing skills which far exceed cognitive skills?
    a. Down syndrome
    b. fragile X syndrome
    c. Williams syndrome
    d. PKU

11. PKU
   a. is more common in males than in females.
   b. is caused by the buildup of an amino acid which is toxic to the nervous system.
   c. is often comorbid with cerebral palsy.
   d. is untreatable.

12. What are teratogens?
   a. substances that cross the placenta during pregnancy and damage the fetus
   b. amino acids which buildup in the body and damage the nervous system
   c. a new group of drugs which are used to treat some forms of mental retardation
   d. small areas of damage caused by physical trauma to the brain

13. Which one of the following statements about the relationship of the environment and the development of mild retardation is false?
   a. The term cultural-familial is used to describe mental retardation without known organic cause.
   b. The effects are usually confined to the mild range of retardation.
   c. Many researchers are focusing on conditions where parents have limited intellectual skills or little education.
   d. There are no intervention programs at the present time which are designed to combat the effects of environmental deprivation.

14. Most programs for treating mental retardation
   a. focus their energy on finding a cure.
   b. rely on medications to control behavior.
   c. attempt to maximize developmental progress, reduce problematic behaviors and help families adjust.
   d. are designed around institutional settings.

15. A commonly used and relatively effective technique designed to increase desired adaptive skills and decrease destructive behavior is
   a. use of medication.
   b. genetic counseling.
   c. behavior modification.
   d. Project Head Start.

Answers to test your understanding

1.	c.	(4-1)
2.	a.	(4-1)
3.	b.	(4-1)
4.	c.	(4-1)
5.	d.	(4-2)
6.	b.	(4-3)
7.	d.	(4-3)
8.	a.	(4-4)
9.	c.	(4-4)
10.	c.	(4-4)
11.	b.	(4-4)
12.	a.	(4-5)
13.	d.	(4-6)(4-7)
14.	c.	(4-8)
15.	c.	(4-8)

| 4-9 | What is autism? |

21. a. Behaviors which are characteristic of autism fall into three general categories. Please list them.

    1.

    2.

    3.

    b. Autism is sometimes described as a _____ (categorical / spectrum) disorder. At one end is typical autism, which is marked by disturbances in _____ (one / two / all) of the above characteristics. At the other end are incomplete or _____ (atypical / pervasive) presentations of the full syndrome.

| 4-10 | What are the features of autism in its typical form? |

22. In your own words, further describe and / or give examples for each of the following general characteristics of autism.

    a. problems with social relationships

    b. expressive language deficits

    c. repetitive or stereotypic behavior

23. a.   In what ways do autism and mental retardation overlap?

    b.   How are autism and mental retardation different?

4-11   What factors influence the development of autism in its typical form?

---

24. We do not fully understand the causes of autism, but researchers are presently looking into a number of possible contributing factors. What evidence supports each of the following views?

    a.   Some cases of autism may be genetically inherited.

    b.   Autism may result from brain damage.

    c.   Autism may result from structural or functional abnormalities of the brain.

25. In order to better understand autism, we must focus on the primary psychological or cognitive deficit which produces the disorder. These deficits may include:

    a.

    b.

    c.

d.

e.

| 4-12 | What are some of the atypical forms of autism? |

26. Asperger's disorder is similar to autism, except that those who suffer with Asperger's disorder have _____ (lower / higher) intellectual skills and normal or near-normal _____ (expressive language / fine motor skills). When compared with individuals with typical autism, people with Asperger's disorder show_____ (less / greater) interest in others.

27. Rett's disorder is much _____ (more / less) common than autism and occurs almost exclusively in _____ (males / females). It appears rather suddenly between _____ (6-18 months / 6-18 years) of age and affects language and motor skills.

| 4-13 | How are pervasive developmental disorders treated? |

28. In your own words, summarize the present status of the treatment of autism and other pervasive developmental disorders, including the different types of treatment and their effectiveness.

| 4-14 | How are learning disabilities defined and identified? |

29. If the term learning disabilities has been around since the 1960's, why has it been so difficult to develop a simple, universally accepted definition?

30. How does the DSM-IV define learning disorder?

4-15	What factors influence the development of reading disabilities?

31. Reading disabilities, often called _____ (phonetic dysfunctional disorders / dyslexia), are the _____ (least / most) frequent learning problem, accounting for about _____ (15-20 percent / 80 percent) of learning disabilities in schools in the United States. The most consistent differences between good and poor readers are _____ (linguistic / perceptual) and it is believed that some reading disabilities may be due to an impaired ability to decipher and effectively use the smallest sound units of language called _____ (auditory bits / phonemes).

32. In your own words, briefly summarize how each of the following may play a role in the development of reading disabilities.

   a. genetic factors

   b. neurological factors

   c. the schools

   d. parents

4-16	How are learning disabilities and reading problems treated?

33. _____ (Medication / Educational intervention) has been the most effective intervention for the treatment of academic deficiencies such as reading disorder. It is believed that a critical period exists between the ages of _____ (5-7 / 15-17) in which reading and writing skills are most easily learned. At the present, reading instruction methods often emphasize _____ (phonic / perceptual) and _____ (meaning / group) based instruction.

Test your understanding

1. Which of the following is not one of the three characteristics of autism?
    a. severe deficits in establishing reciprocal social relationships
    b. nonexistent or poor language skills
    c. almost always comorbid with separation anxiety disorder
    d. stereotyped patterns of behavior, activities or interests

2. Which of the following statements about autism is false?
    a. Autism is more common in males than in females.
    b. Autism is noticeable at an early age.
    c. Autism is commonly comorbid with mental retardation.
    d. Autism is highly treatable if detected soon enough.

3. Autism is often described as a spectrum disorder. This means that
    a. it is commonly treated with drugs.
    b. the effects typically lessen as the child grows into adulthood.
    c. at one end of the spectrum, cases include all three of the typical characteristics of autism and at the other end one finds incomplete presentations.
    d. there are no typical cases of autism.

4. Autism and mental retardation are different in that
    a. children with mental retardation rarely show deficits in language development which is common in autism.
    b. children with mental retardation usually engage others socially whatever language they possess.
    c. autism rarely affects motor skills, which is common in retardation.
    d. autism is much more treatable than mental retardation.

5. Autism
    a. is not related to genetic factors.
    b. is, in almost all cases, caused by abnormalities in brain structure and function.
    c. is better understood today than it was in the past because psychologists now agree on the specific cognitive deficit which causes the disorder.
    d. is probably the result of multiple genetic, neurological and cognitive factors.

6. Asperger's disorder is similar to typical autism, except that those who suffer from Asperger's disorder have
    a. higher intellectual and fine-motor skills.
    b. higher intellectual skills and normal or near normal expressive language.
    c. lower intellectual and fine-motor skills.
    d. lower intellectual skills and greater deficits in expressive language.

7. Rett's disorder occurs almost exclusively in
    a. males.
    b. females.
    c. adolescents with cerebral palsy.
    d. persons with Asperger's disorder.

8. Autism and other pervasive developmental disorders
    a. respond well to various treatments if they are detected soon enough.
    b. respond well to intensive programs stressing intensive education.
    c. are very difficult to treat successfully, although certain aspects of these disorders can be improved with behavior modification.
    d. are very difficult to treat successfully, although certain aspects of these disorders can be improved with medication.

9. The term learning disabilities
    a. is synonymous with the term mental retardation.
    b. is no longer used by educators or psychologists.
    c. is defined by almost all professionals in the field in the same way.
    d. is defined differently by different organizations.

10. According to the DSM-IV, learning disabilities are diagnosed when
    a. IQ is less than 90.
    b. IQ is less than 70.
    c. achievement in reading, writing or mathematics is below that expected for the age, schooling and level of intelligence.
    d. a child has failed more than three different academic subjects in a two year period.

11. Reading disabilities account for approximately _____ percent of learning disabilities in the United States.
    a. 2
    b. 25
    c. 50
    d. 80

12. The most consistent differences between good and poor readers are
    a. linguistic.
    b. perceptual.
    c. hand-eye coordination skills.
    d. based on social class.

13. What is a phoneme?
    a. It is a special telephone used in the education of deaf children.
    b. It is the smallest sound unit of language.
    c. It is a toxin which can cause learning disabilities.
    d. It is the first step in a behavior modification program.

14. The most effective intervention for the treatment of academic deficiencies in schools in the United States has been
    a. stimulant medications for students.
    b. antidepressant medications for teachers.
    c. educational intervention programs.
    d. increased funding for schools.

15. At the present time, reading instruction methods emphasize
    a. phonic and meaning based instruction.
    b. using large groups so that poor readers can model after good readers.
    c. visual exercises needed to improve reading skills.
    d. visual and motor exercises needed to improve reading skills.

Answers to test your understanding

1. c. (4-9)
2. d. (4-9)
3. c. (4-9)
4. b. (4-10)
5. d. (4-10)
6. b. (4-12)
7. b. (4-12)
8. c. (4-13)
9. d. (4-14)
10. c. (4-14)
11. d. (4-15)
12. a. (4-15)
13. b. (4-15)
14. c. (4-16)
15. a. (4-16)

When you have finished . . .

Explore the Web to find more information

An extremely comprehensive Web site for information on mental retardation is **The Arc of the United States** Home Page. (**http://thearc.org/welcome.html**) When you arrive, click on the link <u>Fact Sheets on Topics Related to Mental Retardation</u>.

The Down Syndrome WWW Page is located at (**http://www.nas.com/downsyn/**).

On-Line Asperger's Syndrome Information and Support can be found at their Web site located at (**http://www.udel.edu/bkirby/asperger/**).

The Autism Society of America has an information packed Web site which you can access by going to (**http://www.autism-society.org/**). If you are looking for general information on autism, click on <u>Getting Started (for the newly-diagnosed)</u>.

The **Autism Resources** page (**http://web.syr.edu/~jmwobus/autism/**), which is maintained by John Wobus, has a very large listing of links. The topics include:
> General
> Pages with General Information on Autism
> Other Indexes of Links on Autism
> Online Discussion: mailing lists, etc.
> Asperger's Syndrome
> News
> Accounts
> Bibliography: Books & Articles
> Specific Issues
> Methods, Treatments, Programs
> Academic and Research programs
> Libraries
> Online Papers
> Organizations
> Resources by Language
> For Sale

Internet Mental Health provides a good description of different types of learning disabilities in an article by Larry B. Silver, MD, The Harvard Mental Health Letter, October, 1990. It is located at (**http://www.mentalhealth.com/mag1/p5h-lrn1.html**).

CHAPTER 5
Stress, Sleep, and Adjustment Disorders

Before you read . . .

Survey the chapter

Chapter 5 introduces the concept of stress. It answers the questions of what stress is and how stressful events can affect us both physically and mentally. As you will read, these effects and their causes can vary dramatically from person to person. Why is it that some people seem to be "stress proof" while others seem to be easily incapacitated? What are the major signs of stress and how can one best cope with stressful events?

The chapter begins with the case of Officer Schuler, a police officer in Louisville, Kentucky who, along with her partner, is forced to deal with a brief, but traumatic event, as well as its prolonged aftermath. You will see that the reactions of the two officers to these stressful events, as well as their methods of coping are typical, but quite different.

Following the in depth information about stress and stress management, you will find discussions on two problematic areas which are closely related to stress. The first involves sleep disorders which are disturbances in the quantity or quality of sleep, or unusual behavioral or physiological events which occur during sleep.

The second area discussed is that of adjustment disorders. Although these disorders are frequently diagnosed and the symptoms are relatively mild when compared to many other disorders, they can still significantly interfere with the quality of a person's life, as well as his or her ability to adequately function.

As you read . . .

Ask questions

5-1   What is stress?

5-2   What kinds of events can cause stress?

5-3   Can individual, social or cultural factors affect our reaction to stress-producing events?

5-4   How do psychologists measure stress?

5-5   How do psychologists describe our response to stressors?

5-6   How do researchers describe the psychological reactions of stress?

5-7   How does the immune system work?

5-8   Can prolonged stress negatively affect the immune system?

5-9   How can people cope with stress?

5-10   How are stress and psychological disorders related?

5-11   What is sleep?

5-12   What are sleep disorders?

5-13   What are adjustment disorders?

5-14   What kinds of stressors can cause adjustment disorders?

5-15   How are adjustment disorders treated?

After you read . . .

Review and explore the chapter

5-1   What is stress?

1. Stress is a process that occurs when environmental or social threats called _____ (stress / stressors) place demands on individuals.

2. What three factors affect the way that an individual experiences stress?

    a.

    b.

c.

5-2   What kinds of events can cause stress?

---

3. In your own words, describe or give examples of each of the following categories of potential stressors.

    a.   traumatic events

    b.   predictable stressors

    c.   occupational demands

    d.   relatively minor events (daily hassles)

5-3   Can individual, social or cultural factors affect our reaction to stress-producing events?

---

4. What are three possible explanations for the fact that some people seem to be repeatedly victimized by stressful events?

    a.

    b.

c.

5.   In your own words, briefly describe stressors commonly encountered by each of the following groups.

   a.   members of minority groups

   b.   women

   c.   older persons

6.   It is important to understand that identical stressors affect different individuals in _____ (identical / different) ways. The amount of subjectively perceived stress is _____ (more / less) strongly correlated with later adjustment problems than is the sheer frequency of negative life events.

7.   For each pair of statements below, underline the one that is accurate.

   a.   Unexpected stressors take more of a toll on a person than do predictable ones.

         A stressor is more problematic when the person knows that it is coming and must prepare.

   b.   The negative effect of stressors usually increases when others try to help.

         People usually perceive a stressor as less harmful when they have social support.

   c.   The perceived negative effect of stressors actually decreases when people feel helpless or unable to control the situation.

         The perceived negative effect of stressors dramatically increases when people feel helpless or unable to control the situation.

   d.   A stressor isn't usually as harmful when the person knows that it was caused by the intentional or careless behavior of someone else.

         A stressor is usually perceived as more harmful when the person knows that it was caused by the intentional or careless behavior of someone else.

e.   People who are confident, optimistic and have higher self-esteem tend to be less threatened by stress.

People who are confident, optimistic and have higher self-esteem tend to be more threatened by stress because they're not used to dealing with it.

| 5-4 | How do psychologists measure stress? |

8.   Match the following.

1.   ____ Schedule of Recent Experience
2.   ____ Life Experiences Survey
3.   ____ Hassles Scale

a.   lists fifty-seven items, the respondents themselves rate the positive or negative impact of an event

b.   lists forty-two events, experiences assigned predetermined weight of adaptation and totaled in life change units

c.   focuses on minor everyday stressors which can have a significant cumulative effect

---

| 5-5 | How do psychologists describe our response to stressors? |

9.   Indicate how each of the following statements or examples relate to the stages of Selye's general adaptation syndrome (GAS).

Mark "A " if it describes the alarm stage, "R" for stage of resistance and "E" for stage of exhaustion.

a.   ____ indigestion, loss of weight, insomnia, fatigue, even death

b.   ____ fight or flight response

c.   ____ physical and psychological coping mechanisms

d.   ____ Mrs. Jones's heart starts to race when she hears that she is going to be laid off from her job.

e.   ____ Three weeks later Mrs. Jones feels much calmer. She is sure that she will soon find work.

f.   ____ As the unpaid bills begin to mount, Mrs. Jones's health is deteriorating. She's worried that she might be developing an ulcer.

| 5-6 | How do researchers describe the psychological reactions of stress? |

10. The sympathetic and parasympathetic nervous systems make up the _____ (central / autonomic) nervous system. The _____ (sympathetic / parasympathetic) nervous system works to mobilize the body for fighting and fleeing, while the _____ (sympathetic / parasympathetic) nervous system works to slow down the body's internal functioning.

11. a.   In your own words, briefly describe the chemical process which releases stress hormones during the alarm stage of the stress response.

    b.   In your own words, briefly describe the second process which occurs during the alarm stage which involves the release of catecholamines in the brain.

12. What are endorphins?

13. In your own words, briefly describe the perceptual, cognitive and behavioral adjustments which occur during the alarm stage of the GAS.

| 5-7 | How does the immune system work? |

14. Match the following.

    1.   ____   immune system
    2.   ____   pathogens
    3.   ____   innate immunity
    4.   ____   specific immunity
    5.   ____   macrophages
    6.   ____   interleukins
    7.   ____   T cells
    8.   ____   B cells

        a.   white blood cells which seek out, digest and then spit out pathogens so they can be killed by T cells

b. invading viruses and bacteria

c. present at birth, the first line of defense against pathogens

d. general term for the body's defense network against invading viruses and bacteria

e. release antibodies into the blood to kill pathogens

f. destroy pathogens by deploying chemicals into the cells themselves

g. used by macrophages to summon other immune system defenders such as T cells

h. an acquired defense system which detects the specific type of invading pathogen and destroys it

---

| 5-8 | Can prolonged stress negatively affect the immune system? |

15. a. What is immunosuppression?

b. Why is immunosuppression usually adaptive in the short-run, but potentially costly when maintained over a prolonged period?

| 5-9 | How can people cope with stress? |

16. People's efforts to modify or tolerate stressors is called _____ (coping / the resistence stage).

17. In your own words, briefly describe each of the following coping strategies.

a. problem-focused coping

b. emotion-focused coping

c.   social support

18.   List three possible reasons why persons who enjoy a high level of social support are less likely to suffer from the harmful effects of stress.

a.

b.

c.

Test your understanding

1.   An environmental or social threat that places demands on people is called
      a.   stress.
      b.   a stressor.
      c.   an adjustment demand.
      d.   the alarm stage.

2.   Which of the following is not a common factor which affects the way that an individual experiences stress?
      a.   the nature and timing of the stressors
      b.   the psychological characteristics and social context of the person
      c.   the actual danger posed by the stressor and not the person's perceptions of it
      d.   the biochemical variables that influence the stress response

3.   Which one of the following statements about potential stressors is false?
      a.   Severe traumatic events such as natural disasters, victimization or sudden loss are surprisingly frequent and can leave lasting psychological scars.
      b.   Many potential stressors occur predictably and regularly as a person moves through his or her life. These include marital difficulties, loss of a loved one, etc.
      c.   Some occupations, especially those that make many demands but allow little control, can be particularly stressful.
      d.   In order for an event to be a stressor, it must be traumatic. Daily hassles (arriving late for work or class, losing or breaking something) rarely cause significant stress.

4. The fact that some people seem to be repeatedly victimized by stressful events can be best explained by the fact that (choose two)
    a. some people just have bad luck.
    b. poor social skills or long-term psychological disabilities may increase the chance of unintentionally bringing about stressful events.
    c. one stressor often leads to other stress-producing events.
    d. some persons have a death wish.

5. Older persons
    a. do not handle stress well.
    b. deal with stress better than other social groups.
    c. are more likely to encounter stressors such as economic problems, death of loved ones, chronic illness or loss of physical abilities and attributes.
    d. are much less likely to encounter stressors such as economic problems, death of loved ones, chronic illness or loss of physical abilities and attributes.

6. Which one of the following does not tend to increase the negative effects of stressors?
    a. The stressor is unexpected rather than expected.
    b. The person has the support of others.
    c. The person feels helpless and unable to control the event.
    d. The person feels that the stressor was intentionally caused by another.

7. The psychological scale which asks subjects to rate how much they have been bothered in the prior month by minor problems is the
    a. Schedule of Recent Experiences.
    b. Schedule of Recent Minor Annoyances.
    c. Life Experience Survey.
    d. Hassles Scale.

8. Which of the following occurs in the alarm stage of the General Adaptation Syndrome (GAS)?

    a. fight or flight response
    b. physical and psychological coping mechanisms
    c. weight loss, insomnia, damage to physical health
    d. avoidance, defensive posturing, death

9. Which of the following occurs in the stage of exhaustion of the general adaptation syndrome (GAS)?
    a. fight or flight response
    b. physical and psychological coping mechanisms
    c. weight loss, insomnia, damage to physical health
    d. anger, hostility and aggression

10. Which of the following correctly describes the chemical process which releases stress hormones during the alarm stage?
    a. hypothalamus releases SSS → pituitary releases interleukins → sympathetic system inhibits release of ACTH
    b. hypothalamus produces CRH→ pituitary releases ACTH→ adrenal glands release adrenal corticosteroids → sympathetic nervous system responds
    c. heart rate increases → adrenal glands release adrenalin → sympathetic system responds
    d. hypothalamus releases stress hormones → heart rate decreases → parasympathetic nervous system responds

11. Pathogens are
    a. viruses and bacteria which invade the body.
    b. organs (such as the skin) that are present at birth and are the first line of defense of the immune system.
    c. stress hormones.
    d. white blood cells which seek out, digest and then spit out germs so they can be killed by T cells.

12. Macrophages are
    a. viruses and bacteria which invade the body.
    b. organs (such as the skin) that are present at birth and are the first line of defense of the immune system.
    c. stress hormones.
    d. white blood cells which seek out, digest and then spit out pathogens so they can be killed by T cells.

13. When dealing with prolonged stressors, people often become more susceptible to disease and have slower recovery times. This is due to
    a. the presence of macrophages in the blood.
    b. the suppression of the alarm stage of the GAS.
    c. prolonged immunosuppression.
    d. the fact that sickness is a defense mechanism often used to avoid further stressors.

14. A person's efforts to modify or tolerate stressors is called
    a. coping.
    b. the resistence stage of the GAS.
    c. productive avoidance behavior.
    d. counter immunosuppression.

15. Which of the following was not discussed in the chapter as an effective technique for coping with stress?
    a. problem-focused coping
    b. emotion-focused coping
    c. avoidance-focused coping
    d. social support

Answers to test your understanding

1. b. (5-1)
2. c. (5-1)
3. d. (5-2)
4. b. c. (5-3)
5. c. (5-3)
6. b. (5-3)
7. d. (5-4)
8. a. (5-5)
9. c. (5-5)
10. b. (5-6)
11. a. (5-7)
12. d. (5-7)
13. c. (5-8)
14. a. (5-9)
15. c. (5-9)

5-10	How are stress and psychological disorders related?

19. Each of the following statements is false. Correct each statement to make it true.

    a. Anxiety, helplessness, frustration, hostility, sleeplessness and demoralization are the most common effects of stress. Severe stress however, contributes to one specific mental disorder, posttraumatic stress disorder.

    b. Today, we catagorize physical illnesses which are triggered or worsened by stress, such as heart disease or ulcers, under the heading psychosomatic disorders.

c.   Recent research has shown that the previously held belief that stress may play a role in the onset of depression, bipolar disorder and schizophrenia is unfounded.

d.   The significance of stress for mental disorders was exaggerated by the early versions of the DSM. The DSM-IV has corrected this problem by dropping any reference to stress as a factor relating to mental disorders.

5-11	What is sleep?

20. Match the following.

1. ____ insomnia
2. ____ electroencephalogram (EEG)
3. ____ stage 1 sleep
4. ____ stage 2 sleep
5. ____ stage 3 and 4 sleep
6. ____ rapid eye movement (REM) sleep
7. ____ REM rebound

a   similar to stage 1 sleep, muscle paralysis, dreaming

b.   deep or delta sleep

c.   the first light stage of sleep, it lasts from thirty seconds to ten minutes

d.   measures changes in electrical activity in the brain during sleep

e.   difficulty falling or staying asleep

f.   need to spend more time in REM sleep after periods of REM sleep deprivation

g.   about half of your sleep time is spent in this stage

21. During a night's sleep, most people pass through the full sleep cycle _____ (one or two / four to six) times. Stage 3 and 4 deep sleep occurs in the _____ (first / last) three to five hours of sleep. It is during this time that _____ (dreaming / immune system replenishment) takes place. As the night's sleep continues, more and more time is spent in _____ (stage 3 and 4 deep / stage 2 and REM) sleep where periods of _____ (dreaming / immune system replenishment) occur.

22. a.   What are circadian rhythms?

b.   Where is the location in the brain of the "biological clock"?

c.   What is melatonin?

5-12	What are sleep disorders?

23. Sleep disorders can be a direct result of medical problems, medication or drug abuse. According to the DSM-IV, primary sleep disorders _____ (are / are not) caused by these factors. Primary sleep disorders are divided into two categories. They are disturbances in the amount, quality or timing of a person's sleep, called _____ (dyssomnias / parasomnias) and unusual behaviors or abnormal events during sleep called _____ (dyssomnias / parasomnias).

24. Describe the characteristic features of each of the following dyssomnias.

COMMON DYSSOMNIAS	TYPICAL FEATURES
Primary Insomnia	
Infant Sleep Disturbance (ISD)	
Primary Hypersomnia	
Narcolepsy	
Circadian Rhythm Sleep Disorder	

25. Describe the characteristic features of each of the following parasomnias.

COMMON PARASOMNIAS	TYPICAL FEATURES
Nightmare Disorder	
Sleep Terror Disorder	
Sleepwalking Disorder	

26. What is the most common type of treatment for insomnia and other dyssomnias?

5-13	What are adjustment disorders?

27. A person with adjustment disorder suffers significant behavioral or psychological symptoms in response to _____ (a stressor / the presence of another mental disorder). The symptoms must occur within _____ (three days / three months) after the stressor's appearance and last no longer than _____ (six days / six months) unless the stressor is chronic. Adjustment disorder is very _____ (frequently / rarely) diagnosed and carries _____ (few / many) of the negative stereotypes often associated with other mental disorders.

28. It is usually difficult to differentiate between adjustment disorder and normal reactions to stressors. What criterion is commonly used to make the distinction?

29. What are the two major differences between adjustment disorders and posttraumatic stress disorder?

5-14	What kinds of stressors can cause adjustment disorders?

30. After reading the section, "What Triggers Adjustment Disorders?" in the text, describe an example of this common occurrence from your own life.

| 5-15 | How are adjustment disorders treated? |

31. In your own words, briefly describe the following methods for coping with stressors and the reactions associated with adjustment disorders.

    a.   therapy designed to enhance problem-solving

    b.   therapy designed to enhance emotional coping

    c.   enhancing social support

Test your understanding

1. Today, we categorize physical illnesses which are triggered or worsened by stress as
   a.   psychosomatic disorders.
   b.   psychophysiological disorders.
   c.   Psychological Factors Affecting Medical Condition.
   d.   adjustment disorders.

2. The significance of stress for mental disorders is
   a.   ignored by the DSM-IV.
   b.   opposed by the DSM-IV.
   c.   reflected on Axis III.
   d.   reflected on Axis IV.

3. Dreaming occurs during
   a.   REM sleep.
   b.   NREM sleep.
   c.   stage 2 sleep
   d.   stage 3 and stage 4 sleep

4. The deepest stages of sleep, where immune system and other physical replenishment occurs, are
   a.   REM and NREM sleep.
   b.   stage 1 and stage 2 sleep.
   c.   stage 3 and stage 4 sleep.
   d.   stage 5 and stage 6 sleep.

5. Which category of primary sleep disorders describes disturbances in the amount, quality or timing of a person's sleep?
   a.   the dyssomnias
   b.   the parasomnias
   c.   the sleep-somnias
   d.   insomnia

6. Which category of primary sleep disorders describes unusual or abnormal events during sleep?
   a.   the dyssomnias
   b.   the parasomnias
   c.   the sleep-somnias
   d.   insomnia

7. _____ is a common sleep disorder affecting about one-third of the population, in which the person has trouble falling asleep or staying asleep.
   a. Narcolepsy
   b. Circadian sleep disorder
   c. Primary insomnia
   d. Primary hypersomnia

8. Which of the following sleep disorders describe sudden attacks of REM sleep accompanied by cataplexy?
   a. narcolepsy
   b. circadian sleep disorder
   c. primary insomnia
   d. primary hypersomnia

9. _____ is a sleep disorder most commonly seen in children under age five, in which sleep is interrupted by repeated frightening dreams which occur in REM sleep.
   a. Nightmare disorder
   b. Sleep terror disorder
   c. Sleepwalking disorder
   d. Insomnia

10. Which of the following sleep disorders describe panic and terror occurring in NREM sleep? This disorder is most common in children.
    a. nightmare disorder
    b. sleep terror disorder
    c. sleepwalking disorder
    d. insomnia

11. What is the most common treatment for insomnia and other dyssomnias?
    a. hypnosis
    b. group therapy
    c. REM rebound therapy
    d. medication

12. Adjustment disorders
    a. are very rarely diagnosed.
    b. carry many negative stereotypes compared to other mental disorders.
    c. describe significant behavioral or

psychological symptoms in response to a stressor.
   d. may last for a lifetime.

13. Adjustment disorder is different from the normal reactions to stress because
    a. in adjustment disorder the symptoms of posttraumatic stress disorder are always present.
    b. the person who is suffering from adjustment disorder usually feels as if he or she is handling the stressor adequately.
    c. the person who is suffering from adjustment disorder cannot maintain normal functioning or feels enough distress to seek help.
    d. only in adjustment disorder does the person suffer from physical ailments as a result of the stressor.

14. Situations that cause adjustment disorders
    a. often revolve around marital, academic or occupational setbacks.
    b. are always of long duration.
    c. must reoccur often in a three-month period.
    d. are listed in the DSM-IV.

15. Effective problem solving starts with
    a. identifying possible strategies for a solution.
    b. defining the problem clearly.
    c. removing the stressor from the situation.
    d. finding a good therapist.

Answers to test your understanding

1. c. (5-10)
2. d. (5-10)
3. a. (5-11)
4. c. (5-11)
5. a. (5-12)
6. b. (5-12)
7. c. (5-12)
8. a. (5-12)
9. a. (5-12)
10. b. (5-12)
11. d. (5-12)
12. c. (5-13)
13. c. (5-13)
14. a. (5-14)
15. b. (5-15)

When you have finished . . .

Explore the Web to find more information

Columbia-Presbyterian Medical Center provides a document on "Screening for Hypertension."
You will find it at (**http://cait.cpmc.columbia.edu/texts/gcps/gcps008.html**).

A good article on stress management, "Take Control of Your Stress Monsters" is provided by Making Sense, A Resource for Understanding Women's Health Care Issues, **Planned Parenthood/Chicago Area.**
You can access it at (**http://www.ppca.org/stress.html**).

Sleep Net, which promises to have, "Everything you wanted to know about sleep disorders but were too tired to ask," is located at (**http://www.sleepnet.com/**).

Columbia-Presbyterian Medical Center's Sleep Disorders Center has an informative page which you will find at (**http://cpmcnet.columbia.edu/dept/sleep/slpd0000.html**).

America's House Call Network has a page devoted to sleep disorders information. The URL is
(**http://www.housecall.com/forums/sleep.forum.html**).

Columbia-Presbyterian Medical Center provides the document, "Screening for Abnormal Bereavement."
(**http://cait.cpmc.columbia.edu/texts/gcps/gcps048.html**).

CHAPTER 6
Psychological Factors and Health

Before you read . . .

Survey the chapter

    The last chapter dealt with stress, what it is, what can cause it and how it can affect different people in different ways. Chapter 6 focuses on the relationships between stress, psychological factors which are part of our lives and physical illness.

    The chapter begins with the case of Beth, a 34-year old businessperson and married mother of two small children. Beth is a driven person, constantly pushing herself (and those around her) toward higher and higher goals, while at the same time stifling everyone's growth and achievement. As with so many Americans, it is easy to see that Beth's lifestyle, social relationships, personality and physical health seem to be interrelated in increasingly unhealthy and dangerous ways.

    This chapter examines this interrelationship, beginning with a discussion of health psychology. Psychological and social factors which can affect health are closely examined and their role in increasing the risk of developing such problems as cardiovascular disease, AIDS and cancer is presented. The chapter ends with a discussion of the function of health psychology in the prevention and treatment of health problems.

As you read . . .

Ask questions

6-1   What is health psychology?

6-2   How do we classify psychological factors which affect health?

6-3   How are psychological factors linked to physical disorders?

6-4   What is cardiovascular disease?

6-5   Are stress and cardiovascular disease related?

6-6   How can personality characteristics relate to increased stress and cardiovascular disease?

6-7   Can Type A behavior cause coronary heart disease?

6-8   What role do negative emotions play in coronary heart disease?

6-9   Can psychological factors, such as learning, affect immune system functioning?

6-10   How are psychological factors and AIDS connected?

6-11   How are psychological factors and cancer connected?

6-12   Can social factors be related to an increased likelihood of physical illness?

6-13   What role do psychological factors play in recovering from or coping with illness?

6-14   What are effective psychological interventions for cardiovascular disease?

6-15   What are effective psychological interventions for AIDS?

6-16   What are effective psychological interventions for cancer?

6-17   How can health psychologists help to improve patients' compliance with treatment?

6-18   How can health psychologists help to promote health and prevent illness?

After you read . . .

Review and explore the chapter

6-1   What is health psychology?

1. a.   About what proportion of patients visit a physician because of physical symptoms caused by psychological distress?

    b.   About what proportion of patients visit a physician for physical problems that develop largely because of unhealthy behaviors such as smoking, a faulty diet or alcohol and drug abuse?

c.   About what proportion of patients have conditions such as heart trouble or arthritis that are strongly affected by psychological factors?

2.   a.   What is health psychology?

b.   Name four activities of health psychologists.

1.

2.

3.

4.

3.   Health psychology is based on the biophysical model. What does that mean?

4.   Match the following.

1.   ____ Aristotle and Socrates
2.   ____ the Renaissance
3.   ____ Freud and psychoanalysis
4.   ____ Sir William Osler
5.   ____ modern behavioral medicine

a.   19th century physician, generally considered to be the father of modern behavioral medicine

b.   considers psychological factors as potential influences in almost all diseases

c.   period of rise in dualistic view that mind and body are separate domains

d.   ancient Greek philosophers who saw the necessity of treating both mind and body because they are interconnected

e.   theories challenged dualistic thinking in the late 1800's

---

6-2	How do we classify psychological factors which affect health?

5.   In what three ways has the DSM-IV tried to deal with the classification dilemma caused by the close interrelationship between the mind and body?

a.

b.

c.

6.   In your own words, briefly describe each of the following DSM descriptive categories.

a.   Psychological Factors Affecting Medical Condition

b.   Somatoform Disorders

c.   Factitious Disorders

d.   malingering

| 6-3 | How are psychological factors linked to physical disorders? |

7.   In your own words, briefly describe four ways that psychological factors are linked to illness.

a.

b.

c.

d.

| 6-4 | What is cardiovascular disease? |

8.   Evidence for the adverse effects of psychological variables on physical health is particularly _____ (strong / weak) for cardiovascular disease, which includes diseases of the _____ (brain and nervous / heart and circulatory) system. About _____ (one-fourth / one-half) of deaths each year in the United States are the result of cardiovascular disease. Health psychologists have focused on two leading risks, _____ (stress and personality differences / unhealthy lifestyle and genetic predisposition), to explain this relationship.

9.   Match the following.

1.   ____ atherosclerosis
2.   ____ plaques
3.   ____ aneurysm
4.   ____ angina pectoris
5.   ____ myocardial infarction

6.   ____ stroke
7.   ____ essential hypertension

    a.   high blood pressure which is not caused by any obvious organic factor

    b.   supply of blood to heart muscle is cut off (heart attack)

    c.   a bulge in an artery which may rupture

    d.   blood flow to heart is reduced due to plaques in side walls of blood vessels

    e.   periodic chest pain, squeezing or pressing sensations

    f.   brain tissue and function is damaged by loss of blood and oxygen

    g.   build up of cholesterol and other fatty substances in blood vessels

---

6-5	Are stress and cardiovascular disease related?

10. a.   In your own words, describe the experiments done by Stephan Manuck and his colleagues to study the effects of stress on monkey subjects.

    b.   Do these findings apply to humans?

    c.   What are the two important variables which increase the likelihood that stressors will prove more harmful to health?

11.   Which demographic groups suffer higher rates of heart disease and also tend to show higher blood pressure responses to certain stressors?

> 6-6   How can personality characteristics relate to increased stress and cardiovascular disease?

12. Indicate if the following is a typical characteristic of Type A or Type B behavior.

    a.   competitive   Type ____

    b.   concerned with quality of work more than quantity   Type ____

    c.   heightened sense of time urgency   Type ____

    d.   enjoy tasks which call for sustained analysis and concentration   Type ____

    e.   need to maintain control of situations and others   Type ____

    f.   achievement goals put ahead of social interaction   Type ____

13. The most important Type A assessment device is the structured interview. What two components of the person's responses are taken into account in this test?

    a.

    b.

> 6-7   Can Type A behavior cause coronary heart disease?

14. a.   In your own words, briefly describe the structure and findings of the following studies of Type A behavior as a risk factor for CHD.

    1.   Western Collaborative Group Study (WCGS)

    2.   The Farmington Heart Study

b.   Do the findings of the WCGS and Farmington studies prove that being a Type A person means that you are highly likely to suffer a heart attack or other form of CHD? Why?

| 6-8 | What role do negative emotions play in coronary heart disease? |

15. Recent research suggests that some of the negative emotions that are typical of Type A behavior form the major threats to health. What are these negative emotions?

16. Although the picture is still not totally clear, Type A behavior or chronic negative emotions may be linked to CHD because people with these characteristics consistently _____ (overreact physiologically to / avoid) situations that threaten them or make them angry.   In addition, their competitiveness and hostility create _____ (less and less / more and more) opportunities for conflict, to which they then _____ (overreact / avoid). This could put a strain on arteries and _____ (increase / decrease) the chance of damage. Another possibility could be that frequent angry outbursts or other negative emotions may be accompanied by _____ (a drop in the availability of / rapid swings in) the levels of stress hormones, causing chemical changes which _____ (weaken / harden) the arteries.

Test your understanding

1.   About _____ of patients visit physicians for physical problems that develop largely because of unhealthy behaviors such as smoking, faulty diet or alcohol and drug abuse?
a.   one-tenth
b.   one-fifth
c.   one-third
d.   one-half

2.   Which of the following is not an important activity of health psychologists?
a.   understanding how psychological and physiological factors interact to influence illness and health
b.   identifying risk factors for sickness, as well as protective factors for health
c.   developing and implementing programs designed to promote the belief that mind and body functions are separate but equal
d.   developing and implementing techniques for promoting healthy behaviors

3.   Modern behavioral medicine
a.   considers psychological factors as potential influences in almost all diseases.
b.   promotes a dualistic view that mind and body are separate domains.
c.   is composed of physicians dedicated to the treatment of behavioral disorders.
d.   is composed of physicians dedicated to the improvement and enhancement of the behavior of doctors and other medical professionals.

4. Which of the following is not one of the ways that the DSM-IV has tried to deal with the classification dilemma caused by the close interrelationship between mind and body?
   a. Axis III concentrates on general medical conditions that are related to medical disorder.
   b. The DSM-IV provides special rules for classifying mental disorders caused by drugs and medical conditions.
   c. The DSM directs clinicians to use multiple diagnoses to classify all the conditions that might apply to a patient.
   d. Axis VI has been dropped.

5. The DSM descriptive category, Psychological Factors Affecting Medical Condition, describes
   a. situations in which psychological factors have contributed to actual physical damage to the body.
   b. situations in which a person complains of physical symptoms, but there is no diagnosable physical reason to account for those symptoms.
   c. situations in which a person is intentionally faking or exaggerating physical symptoms in order to play the sick role.
   d. situations in which a person is intentionally faking or exaggerating physical symptoms for a reason other than psychological gain.

6. Which of the following statements about the interrelationship of psychological factors and illness is false?
   a. Disease can cause psychological changes such as feelings of depression.
   b. The development of disease is influenced by underlying biological influences, while psychological conditions are influenced by underlying cognitive processes.

   c. Psychological and social influences may exert a direct influence on biological processes that, in turn, are implicated in the cause of disease.
   d. Psychological and social influences may indirectly lead to disease because they are associated with unhealthy behaviors.

7. Health psychologists have focused on which two risk factors to explain the relationship between CHD and psychological factors?
   a. unhealthy life styles and genetic predisposition
   b. angina pectoris and myocardial infarction
   c. stress and personality differences
   d. socioeconomic status (SES) and age

8. What is atherosclerosis?
   a. high blood pressure which is not caused by any obvious organic factor
   b. when the supply of blood to heart muscle is cut off (heart attack)
   c. when the blood flow to the heart is reduced due to plaques in side walls of blood vessels
   d. periodic chest pain, squeezing or pressing sensations

9. Two especially important variables which increase the likelihood that stressors will have a harmful effect on health are (1) if they are chronic and (2)
   a. if they exceed the person's perceived ability to cope.
   b. if they involve social relationships.
   c. if they are not treated immediately by a health psychologist.
   d. if they are not treated immediately by a physician.

10. Which of the following demographic groups suffer higher rates of heart disease and also tend to show higher blood pressure responses to certain stressors?

a.   White Americans, women and adolescents
b.   Asian Americans, men and middle-aged persons
c.   Hispanic Americans, women and children
d.   Black Americans, men and older persons

11. Sarah is a hard driving, competitive businessperson. She is always in a hurry and often becomes hostile and angry when she can't control a situation. Sarah is best described as
a.   a Type A person.
b.   a Type B person.
c.   a Type C person.
d.   a person who definitely will have a heart attack someday.

12. Joe is a businessperson who is easygoing and unhurried, uncompetitive and concerned more with the quality of his work than the quantity. Joe can best be described as
a.   a Type A person.
b.   a Type B person.
c.   a Type C person.
d.   a person who definitely will never have a heart attack.

13. Which statement about Type A personality characteristics is true?
a.   Studies consistently show that Type A behavior causes CHD and associated heart attacks.
b.   Studies consistently show that Type B, not A, is the true cause of CHD.
c.   Even though studies have shown that Type A persons may have higher rates of CHD when compared to Type B's, the vast majority of Type A's never develop CHD.
d.   No study has ever found a relationship between Type A personality characteristics and CHD.

14. Recent research suggests that the Type A characteristics most likely linked to CHD are
a.   avoidance and fear, especially of persons in control.
b.   hostility, especially when it involves cynicism and chronic suspiciousness and anger.
c.   competitiveness and the lack of feeling of success.
d.   lack of sleep and a poor diet caused by constant hurry and hyperactivity.

15. Possible reasons why Type A behavior and negative emotions may br linked to CHD include all of the following except
a.   Type A behavior and negative emotions cause people to overreact to situations, which if chronic, can strain arteries causing damage.
b.   chronic Type A behavior and negative emotions increase the opportunity for conflict and further overarousal.
c.   frequent angry outbursts and other negative emotions may be accompanied by rapid swings in the level of stress hormones, which can cause cardiovascular damage.
d.   frequent angry outbursts and other negative emotions may actually increase immune system functioning so much that necessary energy is taken away from the cardiovascular system.

Answers to test your understanding

1.	c.	(6-1)
2.	c.	(6-1)
3.	a.	(6-1)
4.	d.	(6-2)
5.	a.	(6-2)
6.	b.	(6-3)

7. c. (6-4)
8. c. (6-4)
9. a. (6-5)
10. d. (6-5)
11. a. (6-6)
12. b. (6-6)
13. c. (6-7)
14. b. (6-8)
15. d. (6-8)

6-9   Can psychological factors, such as learning, affect immune system functioning?

17. a. What is anticipatory nausea?

    b. What is the most likely explanation for anticipatory nausea?

    c. What psychological techniques are used to treat anticipatory nausea?

6-10   How are psychological factors and AIDS connected?

18. Answer the questions in the table below.

ACQUIRED IMMUNE DEFICIENCY SYNDROME (AIDS)	
What are the specific effects of HIV on the immune system?	
What are the secondary effects of HIV on body function?	

Why is HIV difficult to control with drug therapy?	
How is HIV transmitted?	
How many people are HIV positive in the world today?	
Which two groups have the largest number of AIDS cases in the U. S. today? By the year 2000?	
HIV infections are increasing rapidly in which groups in the U.S. today?	

19. a.   Describe how the following psychological /behavioral factors are implicated in AIDS.

    1.   high-risk sexual behaviors

    2.   intravenous drug use

    b.   What is another way that psychological factors may influence the overall course of AIDS?

6-11   How are psychological factors and cancer connected?

20. Normally, cells in the body divide in a _____ (random / orderly) way, directed by the right match of _____ (proteins and protein / hormones and hormone) receptors. When cells reproduce wildly with no direction, _____ (a tumor / death) results. Cancer is actually a collection of diseases that begins with a malfunction in the way DNA _____ (is produced in the body /

controls cell growth). One out of every _____ (three / thirty) Americans will be diagnosed with some form of cancer in his or her lifetime.

21. What are three ways in which cancer may be linked to psychological factors?

   a.

   b.

   c.

6-12   Can social factors be related to an increased likelihood of physical illness?

---

22. In your own words, briefly describe how each of the following attempts to explain the fact that the lower a person's socioeconomic status (SES), the greater one's chance of illness and premature death.

   a.   social drift hypothesis

   b.   biochemical processes

   c.   psychological characteristics (negative emotions)

   d.   stressors

   e.   unhealthy behaviors

6-13   What role do psychological factors play in recovering from or coping with illness?

---

23. In general, the most effective interventions of behavioral medicine employ a package of three different components. Briefly describe each.

a.

b.

c.

6-14   What are effective psychological interventions for cardiovascular disease?

---

24. a.   What behaviors are commonly targeted for change to help reduce risk factors for CHD?

b.   Can Type A behaviors be changed? How? Is it an effective way to reduce the reoccurrence of heart attacks?

6-15   What are effective psychological interventions for AIDS?

---

25. In your own words, briefly discuss different AIDS prevention programs both in the United States and in other parts of the world.

26. In your own words, briefly describe those psychological interventions which are designed to help patients cope with HIV/AIDS itself.

| 6-16 | What are effective psychological interventions for cancer? |

27. a.   In your own words, briefly describe how psychological interventions have been used to improve the psychological and physical well-being of cancer patients.

    b.   Are behaviorally oriented psychotherapies effective ways of preventing cancer and prolonging the lives of cancer patients?

| 6-17 | How can health psychologists help to improve patients' compliance with treatment? |

28.   Whether a prescribed treatment for a medical illness is effective depends on two basic factors. First, the treatment needs to be _____ (affordable / correct). Second, the patient need to follow through with the treatment. This is called _____ (compliance / self-care).

29. a.   Systematic attempts to increase patient compliance fall into three categories. What are they?

        1.

        2.

        3.

    b.   In your own words, briefly describe and give examples for each of the following cognitive-behavioral techniques commonly used to increase patient compliance.

        1.   use of environmental cues

   2.   use of contingency contracts

   3.   token economies

   4.   behavioral therapy to reduce side effects

6-18	How can health psychologists help to promote health and prevent illness?

30. The text states that we can try to promote health and prevent illness by helping people break unhealthy health practices, which are responsible for about half of the deaths in the United States each year. What are those behavioral risk factors?

   a.

   b.

   c.

   d.

   e.

f.

31. a.   We can promote good physical health by helping people develop and maintain good health habits. List four examples of healthy behaviors below.

1.

2.

3.

4.

b.   What are some of the reasons that health-promotion efforts are not completely successful?

32. In your own words, briefly describe the health belief model (HBM).

Test your understanding

1. What is anticipatory nausea?
   a. It is a symptom of cancer.
   b. In cancer patients, it is nausea and vomiting occurring in the 12-hour period preceding chemotherapy.
   c. In cancer patients, it is nausea and vomiting occurring in the 12-hour period after chemotherapy, when the patient anticipates the next session.
   d. It is an early warning sign of CHD.

2. What causes anticipatory nausea?
   a. learning
   b. low socioeconomic status
   c. plaque buildup on the walls of arteries
   d. hormonal changes due to over medication

3. What is the effect of HIV on the immune system?
   a. HIV causes a rapid increase of T cells.
   b. HIV destroys T cells.
   c. HIV replaces T cells with HIV cells.
   d. HIV replaces T cells with AIDS cells.

4. HIV infections are increasing especially rapidly in which groups in the United States?
   a. older, high income, Black and Hispanic American men
   b. low income, White American adolescents and young men
   c. older, high income, White American men
   d. young women, low income Black and Hispanic American adolescents

5. Cancer is
   a. for the most part learned, according to health psychologists.
   b. not a leading cause of death in the United States.
   c. actually a collection of diseases that begins with a malfunction in the way DNA controls cell growth.
   d. most influenced in both development and treatment by the so called Type C behavior pattern.

6. Which of the following is not one of the ways that cancer may be linked to psychological and social factors?
   a. The incidence of cancer in the United States is mildly linked to ethnicity and gender.
   b. Unhealthy behavioral habits, such as smoking or eating fatty foods, increase the risk of several types of cancer.
   c. Some studies indicate a Type C, cancer prone personality.
   d. Some types of cancer are now successfully treated with only cognitive-behavioral and group therapy.

7. Is there a relationship between a person's socioeconomic status (SES) and the chance of illness and premature death?
   a. No.
   b. Yes. The lower one's SES, the lower the incidence of illness and premature death.
   c. Yes. The lower one's SES, the higher the incidence of illness and premature death.
   d. Yes. The higher one's SES, the higher the incidence of illness and premature death.

8. In general, the most effective interventions of behavioral medicine
   a. are based on finding the right medication.
   b. are based on one thing, social support.
   c. are focused around traditional psychoanalytic psychotherapy and biofeedback.
   d. employ a combination of stress reduction techniques, cognitive restructuring and social support.

9. Can Type A behavior be changed?
   a. Yes. Type A behavior can be altered to a certain extent with counseling.
   b. Yes. Type A behavior can be changed, but only if the person has already had a heart attack.
   c. No. Only Type B behavior can be altered.
   d. No. Neither Type A nor Type B behavior can be changed.

10. AIDS prevention programs, both in the United States and in other parts of the world, include all of the following except
    a. programs which include education, skills training and group support.
    b. spraying programs designed to kill the virus which causes AIDS.
    c. clean needle exchange and condom distribution programs.
    d. programs designed to empower women.

11. Which two of the following have been shown to occur as a result of individual, group and behavioral therapy with cancer patients?
    a. Patient distress levels are reduced.
    b. Almost 80 percent of patients are in remission from their cancer within six months of beginning the therapy.
    c. Immune system functioning improves and reoccurrence rates decrease.
    d. Anticipatory nausea disappears.

12. How well patients follow through with their medical treatment plans is called
    a. the patient responsibility factor.
    b. patient compliance.
    c. self-care.
    d. self-directed health care.

13. All of the following are common methods used to increase patient compliance except
    a. educating the patient about the importance of compliance, so that he or she will take a more active role in maintaining his or her own health.
    b. modifying the treatment plan so that it

is easier to comply.
    c. using behavioral and cognitive-behavioral techniques to increase the patient's ability to stay in medical compliance.
    d. discontinuing treatment periodically in order to avoid patient burnout.

14. Unhealthy practices such as faulty eating habits, failure to use seatbelts, failure to obtain and comply with medical treatment, engaging in risky sexual behaviors and abusing tobacco, alcohol and illegal drugs are responsible for _____ percent of all deaths in the United States each year.
    a. ten
    b. twenty-five
    c. fifty
    d. ninety

15. Which of the following is not a major component of the health belief model?
    a. Compliance is affected by how the person perceives the seriousness of the illness and their susceptibility to it.
    b. Compliance is affected by how effective the treatment is when compared to how costly or difficult the patient perceives it to be.
    c. Compliance is affected by how motivated the patient is by internal cues (for example pain) or external factors.
    d. Compliance is most affected by the patient's perception of the illness and this is determined for the most part by the "bedside manner" of the doctor.

Answers to test your understanding

1. b. (6-9)
2. a. (6-9)
3. b. (6-10)
4. d. (6-10)
5. c. (6-11)
6. d. (6-11)
7. c. (6-12)
8. d. (6-13)
9. a. (6-14)
10. b. (6-15)
11. a. c. (6-16)
12. b. (6-17)
13. d. (6-17)
14. c. (6-18)
15. d. (6-18)

When you have finished . . .

Explore the Web to find more information

The Centers for Disease Control and Prevention has a Web site with information and links. Their home page is located at (http://www.cdc.gov/). When you get there, click on Health Information.

Cornell University Medical College provides an in depth document, "Normal Immune System," at (http://edcenter.med.cornell.edu/CUMC_PathNotes/Immunopathology/Immuno_01.html).

National Institutes of Health Publication No. 96-3412, "Spread the Word about Cancer: A Guide for Black Americans," is located at (http://www.pueblo.gsa.gov/cic_text/health/cncrblak.txt).

The document, "Psychosocial Aspects of AIDS, January 1992 through May 1994, 1275 Citations," prepared by Peggie S. Tillman, Ph.D., M.L.S., **National Library of Medicine** and Edward R. Turner, M.S.W., **National Institutes of Mental Health**, can be accessed by going to (gopher://gopher.nlm.nih.gov:70/00/bibs/cbm/psycaids.txt).

"Women & AIDS," a reprint from FDA Consumer Magazine (1993) can be located at (http://www.pueblo.gsa.gov/cic_text/health/other/womeaids.txt).

A number of interesting articles on health interventions from **Columbia Presbyterian Medical Center** are available on the Web.

- "Counseling to Prevent Tobacco Use"
  (**http://cait.cpmc.columbia.edu/texts/gcps/gcps053.html**)

- "Screening for Infection with Human Immunodeficiency Virus"
  (**http://cait.cpmc.columbia.edu/texts/gcps/gcps029.html**)

- "Counseling to Prevent HIV and Other Sexually Transmitted Diseases"
  (**http://cait.cpmc.columbia.edu/texts/gcps/gcps058.html**)

- "Counseling to Prevent Motor Vehicle Injuries"
  (**http://cait.cpmc.columbia.edu/texts/gcps/gcps056.html**)

- "Counseling to Prevent Household and Environmental Injuries"
  (**http://cait.cpmc.columbia.edu/texts/gcps/gcps057.html**)

CHAPTER 7
Anxiety Disorders

Before you read . . .

Survey the chapter

Chapter 7 begins with the case of Jim, a forty year old who goes through a life threatening traumatic event which is so overwhelming that anyone would experience intense anxiety and fear. Even though the event itself is short lived, for Jim, the anxiety and depression associated with it are not. Eight years later, though he is physically healed, he remains emotionally scarred.

Jim is suffering from posttraumatic stress disorder, one of the eight major anxiety disorders discussed in this chapter. These different disorders describe different ways that anxiety can disrupt functioning. As you will read, sometimes anxiety is chronic and seemingly unremitting and sometimes it attacks in sudden overwhelming waves. You will read about disorders which describe situations in which intense anxiety is attached to an obvious event, as with Jim, or other disorders where the event is less obvious or perhaps innocent and unthreatening to most people. In any event, you will see that the common underlying issue in each of the disorders described in this chapter is anxiety which has gone awry.

As you read . . .

Ask questions

7-1   What is anxiety?

7-2   Are phobic disorders commonly diagnosed?

7-3   What are the typical characteristics of specific phobia?

7-4   What are the typical characteristics of social phobia?

7-5   What factors can cause the development of phobic disorders?

7-6   How are phobic disorders treated?

7-7   What is panic disorder and how is it related to agoraphobia?

7-8   What causes the development of panic disorder and agoraphobia?

7-9   How are panic disorder and agoraphobia treated?

7-10   What is obsessive-compulsive disorder (OCD)?

7-11   What factors can influence the development of OCD?

7-12   How is OCD treated?

7-13   What is generalized anxiety disorder (GAD)?

7-14   What factors cause GAD?

7-15   How is GAD treated?

7-16   What is posttraumatic stress disorder (PTSD)?

7-17   What causes PTSD?

7-18   How is PTSD treated?

After you read . . .

Review and explore the chapter

| 7-1   What is anxiety? |

1. Anxiety disorders are the _____ (least / most) prevalent of all mental disorders in the United States and perhaps throughout _____ (North America / the world). Current research shows that _____ (one-tenth / one-fourth) of American adolescents and adults have experienced one of these disorders and as many as _____ (eight / twenty-eight) million Americans either have had an anxiety disorder in the last year or are currently experiencing one.

2. Both fear and anxiety are expressed in three major ways. What are they?

    a.

b.

c.

3.   In what ways are anxiety and fear different from each other?

4.   a.   What is a neurosis?

     b.   Is the concept of neurosis used as an official diagnosis in the DSM-IV?

5.   How is anxiety viewed today?

7-2   Are phobic disorders commonly diagnosed?

---

6.   A phobia is _____ (a rational / an irrational), _____ , (annoying / excessive) fear that causes intense emotional distress and _____ (mild inconvenience in / significantly interferes with) everyday life.

7.   a.   Would phobias best be categorized as a commonly diagnosed or rarely diagnosed mental disorder?

     b.   Phobias are more commonly diagnosed in which gender and ethnic groups in the United States?

7-3   What are the typical characteristics of specific phobia?

---

8.   Specific phobias involve intense, persistent fear of specific _____ (objects or situations / violent acts) that objectively pose _____ (little or no / extreme) threat to the person.

9.   Both of the statements below about specific phobia are false. Correct both statements to make them true.

   a.   According to the DSM-IV criteria for specific phobia, extreme distress occurs only when the person is directly exposed to the feared situation.

   b.   In order to meet the DSM-IV criteria for specific phobia, the intensity level of the anxiety need only create enough cognitive distress so that the person is concerned.

10. In your own words, briefly describe each of the following common categories of specific phobia.

   a.   animal phobias

   b.   blood, injections and injury phobias

   c.   situational phobias

7-4   What are the typical characteristics of social phobia?

---

11. Social phobias involve an excessive fear of situations in which the person might be _____ (attacked / evaluated) and possibly _____ (killed / embarrassed).

12. a. Describe some of the most commons situations which induce social phobias.

    b. What are generalized social phobias and why are generalized social phobias more disruptive to a person's life?

7-5   What factors can cause the development of phobic disorders?

13. In your own words, briefly summarize each of the following attempts to explain the causes of phobic disorder.

    a. the psychoanalytic view

    b. behavioral and cognitive factors

    c. biological theories

    d. preparedness theory

7-6   How are phobic disorders treated?

14. Match the following.

    1. ____ systematic desensitization
    2. ____ anxiety hierarchy
    3. ____ in vivo situations
    4. ____ graduated exposure
    5. ____ flooding

6. ____ modeling
7. ____ participant modeling
8. ____ self-efficacy

    a.   immediate and prolonged presentation of the most intense version of the feared stimulus

    b.   clients experience live, rather than imagined, exposure to items from an anxiety hierarchy

    c.   a live situation

    d.   a graduated list of fear provoking stimuli ranging from least to most threatening

    e.   a combination of in vivo exposure and modeling

    f.   therapeutic process of successive gradual exposure to items on an anxiety hierarchy while remaining relaxed and calm

    g.   repeated observation of others fearlessly engaging in phobic situation

    h.   perhaps the common element in all of the different treatments for phobic disorder, the belief of the patient that they can approach and tolerate their feared situations or objects

---

7-7	What is panic disorder and how is it related to agoraphobia?

15. Panic disorder consists of periodic and unexpected attacks of intense, terrifying anxiety called _____ (panic attacks / agoraphobia). The attacks come on _____ (suddenly / slowly) and may last a few _____ (minutes or hours / days or weeks). The person often develops persistent anxiety that _____ (they will die or go crazy / other attacks will occur).

16. a.   In your own words, briefly describe agoraphobia.

    b.   Why are panic disorder and agoraphobia often seen together?

    c.   Persons displaying panic disorder with agoraphobia are vulnerable to other problems. What are they?

7-8	What causes the development of panic disorder and agoraphobia?

17. In your own words, briefly summarize each of the following attempts to explain the causes of panic disorder and agoraphobia.

    a.   psychoanalytic theory

    b.   biological factors

    c.   diathesis-stress models

7-9	How are panic disorder and agoraphobia treated?

18. a.   Cognitive-behavioral treatment is based on a specific assumption. What is it?

    b.   Cognitive-behavioral treatment typically contains three basic elements. List and briefly describe these elements below.

       1.

       2.

       3.

c. Are cognitive-behavioral techniques generally effective in eliminating panic attacks?

d. In your own words, briefly describe panic-control treatment as an intervention in anxiety disorders.

19. Which types of medications are commonly used to treat panic disorder? Have they proven to be effective?

Test your understanding

1. Which category of mental disorders are the most prevalent in the United States and perhaps the world?
    a. the somatoform disorders
    b. schizophrenia
    c. the anxiety disorders
    d. phobic disorders

2. Anxiety and fear are commonly expressed in which three common ways?
    a. cognitive distress, physiological arousal, and behavioral disruption and avoidance
    b. hallucinations, delusions, nightmares
    c. nightmares, sleep loss, behavioral disruption and avoidance
    d. worry, physiological arousal, stress

3. Are fear and anxiety different from each other?
    a. No, fear and anxiety are the same thing.
    b. Yes, fear refers to a response to a specific perceived danger, while anxiety is usually used to describe a more vague sense of apprehension that something threatening may occur.

c. Yes, anxiety refers to a response to a specific perceived danger, while fear is usually used to describe a more vague sense of apprehension that something threatening may occur.
d. Yes, anxiety is always a symptom of mental disorder, while fear is a normal behavior.

4. A phobia can best be described as
    a. any excessive fear.
    b. any excessive fear which interferes with daily life.
    c. an irrational fear.
    d. an irrational, excessive fear which interferes with daily life.

5. Statistically, which of the following groups would have the lowest rates of phobic disorders?
    a. White men
    b. White women
    c. Black Americans
    d. Hispanics

6. Which of the following statements about specific phobia is false?
   a. Specific phobia involves intense, persistent fear of specific objects or situations that objectively pose little or no threat to the person.
   b. In specific phobia, the distress often occurs not only with direct exposure, but also when the person anticipates exposure to the feared situation.
   c. In order to meet the DSM-IV criteria for specific phobia, the fear must be intense enough to interfere significantly with the person's life.
   d. The most common category of specific phobia is a fear of using public restrooms or other possibly humiliating social situations.

7. Which category of phobic disorder involves an excessive fear of situations in which the person might be evaluated and possibly embarrassed?
   a. specific phobia
   b. social phobia
   c. agoraphobia
   d. situational phobia

8. The preparedness theory of phobic disorders assumes that phobias can be caused by
   a. unresolved conflicts and repressed sexual urges.
   b. learning.
   c. too much of the neurotransmitter GABA in the brain.
   d. the idea that some persons may be "prewired" to overreact to certain types of stimuli.

9. A graduated list of fear producing stimuli which is commonly used in the treatment of phobic disorders is called
   a. the in vivo list.
   b. an anxiety hierarchy.
   c. the modeling plan.
   d. the desensitization layout.

10. An in vivo situation is
    a. a live situation.
    b. an imagined situation.
    c. the content from a drug induced dream.
    d. the content from a nightmare.

11. How long do panic attacks last?
    a. They usually last for a few seconds.
    b. They usually last for a few minutes.
    c. They usually last for a few weeks.
    d. Panic attacks are constant and ongoing, often for years at a time.

12. Are agoraphobia and panic disorder often seen together?
    a. No, because it is impossible for a person to show symptoms of agoraphobia and have panic attacks at the same time.
    b. No, because agoraphobia is only seen in children under the age of eighteen, while panic disorder occurs only in adults.
    c. Yes, because agoraphobia often develops from a history of panic attacks.
    d. Yes, because according to the DSM-IV, agoraphobia and panic disorder have the same symptoms.

13. Panic disorder and agoraphobia
    a. tend to run in families, which suggests a genetic component.
    b. are probably not related to genetic factors, because they have different symptoms.
    c. have been shown by researchers to be totally learned behaviors, which are not influenced by biological factors.
    d. have been shown by researchers to be caused by unlearned biological alarms which create anxious apprehension.

14. Which of the following is not one of the basic elements typically seen in cognitive-behavioral treatment of panic disorder and agoraphobia?
    a.   breathing retraining
    b.   interoceptive exposure to somatic cues which trigger attacks
    c.   drug therapy
    d.   cognitive restructuring

15. Which types of medications are commonly used to treat panic disorder?
    a.   antidepressants only
    b.   antidepressants and antianxiety agents such as the benzodiazepines
    c.   depressants and tranquilizers
    d.   Panic disorder is rarely treated with medications, because none have proven to be useful.

Answers to test your understanding

1.	c.	(7-1)
2.	a.	(7-1)
3.	b.	(7-1)
4.	d.	(7-2)
5.	a.	(7-2)
6.	d.	(7-3)
7.	b.	(7-4)
8.	d.	(7-5)
9.	b.	(7-6)
10.	a.	(7-6)
11.	b.	(7-7)
12.	c.	(7-7)
13.	a.	(7-8)
14.	c.	(7-9)
15.	b.	(7-9)

7-10	What is obsessive-compulsive disorder (OCD)?

20. a.   In your own words, describe what clinicians are referring to when they use the term obsession when describing OCD.

    b.   How does this use of the term obsession differ from the common use of the term to describe a person obsessed with, for example, a romantic partner or a sports activity, or a person who described as a compulsive eater or compulsive gambler?

21. In your own words, describe what clinicians are referring to when they use the term compulsion when describing OCD.

22. Mark the following with the letter O if it is an example of an obsession. Use the letter C if it is an example of a compulsion.

   a.   ____   Megan consistently worries that she has injured someone.

   b.   ____   Ramos washes his hands over fifty times a day.

   c.   ____   Rebecca can't seem to get out of her mind the idea that her hands are dirty.

   d.   ____   William must count the ceiling tiles in his kitchen before he can leave the room.

23. In your own words, briefly describe Tourette's disorder.

| 7-11 | What factors can influence the development of OCD? |

24. In your own words, briefly summarize each of the following attempts to explain the causes of obsessive compulsive disorder.

   a.   genetics

   b.   neurological factors

   c.   cognitive-behavioral factors

| 7-12 | How is OCD treated? |

25. In your own words, briefly describe each of the following treatments for obsessive-compulsive disorder.

   a.   cingulotomy

b.   clomipramine

c.   exposure and response prevention

7-13   What is generalized anxiety disorder (GAD)?

26. People with generalized anxiety disorder worry _____ (sporadically / chronically) about _____ (one specific situation / numerous minor events) to the point that the anxiety and worry dominate their lives and interfere with their daily functioning.

27. Circle the social group in each category which has the highest diagnosed rate of GAD.

    a.   men   or   women

    b.   persons under age thirty   or   persons over age thirty

    c.   young Black males   or   older White females

    d.   high socioeconomic status   or   low socioeconomic status

---

7-14   What factors cause GAD?

28. a.   Why are theories about the causes of GAD less well developed than those of other anxiety disorders?

    b.   In your own words, briefly discuss two possible explanations of GAD from a psychological perspective.

       1.

       2.

| 7-15 | How is GAD treated? |

29. In your own words, briefly describe each of the following treatments for generalized anxiety disorder.

    a.   cognitive-behavioral treatment

    b.   drug treatments

| 7-16 | What is posttraumatic stress disorder (PTSD)? |

30. The symptoms of posttraumatic stress disorder fall into three broad classes. What are they?

    a.

    b.

    c.

31. According to the DSM-IV, which disorder describes PTSD-like symptoms which occur within one month following a traumatic stressor and last more than two days, but less than one month?

7-17   What causes PTSD?

32. How do each of the following attempt to explain the fact that some persons experience extreme trauma and remain symptom free, while others develop the symptoms of PTSD?

   a.   characteristics of the trauma itself

   b.   what happens to the victim after the trauma

   c.   the personality and stress-coping style of the trauma victim

   d.   biological predisposition

33. In your own words, briefly explain how the two factor conditioning model and fear networks theories attempt to explain the development of PTSD symptoms.

   a.   two-factor conditioning

   b.   fear networks

7-18   How is PTSD treated?

34. In your own words, briefly explain how the following are used to treat PTSD.

   a.   direct exposure treatment

b.   cognitive therapies

c.   drug treatments

Test your understanding

1.   Unwanted, disturbing, often irrational thoughts, feelings or images that people cannot get out of their minds are called
a.   obsessions.
b.   compulsions.
c.   hallucinations.
d.   illusions.

2.   Which of the following is an example of a compulsion?
a.   fear of germs and contamination
b.   not being able to leave for class on time because you have to keep checking to make sure that the door is locked
c.   constant worry about injuring others
d.   almost always washing your hands before eating a meal

3.   Which of the following statements about Tourette's disorder is false?
a.   Tourette's disorder is a genetic disorder probably related to OCD.
b.   Tourette's disorder is often comorbid with OCD.
c.   Major symptoms of Tourette's disorder include both motor and verbal tics.
d.   To meet the DSM-IV criteria for Tourette's disorder, the person must display coprolalia (verbal obscenities).

4.   Which of the following is the least likely to be viewed by most clinicians today as a legitimate cause of obsessive-compulsive disorder?

a.   the role of genetic factors which possibly predispose persons to OCD
b.   problems with brain function and structure as a contributing factor in OCD
c.   the fact that OCD is caused by unconscious conflicts and repressed sexual urges
d.   the role of learning in the development of OCD

5.   What is cingulotomy?
a.   It is a rarely used form of psychosurgery, which is successful only in a minority of OCD cases.
b.   It is a very commonly used form of psychosurgery, which is dramatically successful in most OCD cases.
c.   It is a drug commonly used in the treatment of OCD.
d.   It is a complex form of systematic desensitization therapy used in the treatment of OCD.

6.   Generalized anxiety disorder is characterized by
a.   many frequent and persistent panic attacks.
b.   chronic stress caused by a chaotic life.
c.   chronic worry about one specific minor event.
d.   chronic worry about numerous minor events.

7. Statistically, which of the following groups would have the lowest rates of generalized anxiety disorder?
   a. White men, over 30, with higher socioeconomic status
   b. young Black males
   c. persons of low socioeconomic status
   d. young women

8. Theories about the causes of generalized anxiety disorder
   a. are better supported by research than theories for other anxiety disorders.
   b. are less well developed than theories for the other anxiety disorders.
   c. are nonexistent.
   d. are usually tied to genetic factors.

9. Which two of the following best describe possible explanations of GAD from a psychological perspective.
   a. The constant worry seen in GAD is caused by unconscious conflicts and repressed sexual urges.
   b. The constant worry seen in GAD may be an attempt to maintain tight control over all aspects of one's life.
   c. The constant worry seen in GAD is caused by a lack of GABA in the brain.
   d. The constant worry seen in GAD may function as a way to actually avoid emotional or physical feelings of anxiety.

10. Which of the following is not a common treatment for GAD?
    a. drug treatment
    b. cognitive restructuring
    c. psychosurgery
    d. relaxation training

11. Which of the following is not one of the general categories of symptoms of posttraumatic stress disorder?
    a. frequently reexperiencing the event
    b. persistent avoidance of stimuli associated with the event and a general numbing of emotions
    c. increased physiological arousal
    d. increased tolerance of life stressors

12. According to the DSM-IV, which disorder describes PTSD-like symptoms which occur within one month following a traumatic stressor and last more than two days, but less than one month?
    a. PTSD
    b. acute stress disorder
    c. minimal stress disorder
    d. agoraphobia

13. The chances of developing PTSD symptoms following a severe stressor decreases when
    a. the person perceives the situation as overwhelming and uncontrollable.
    b. the person receives social support after the event.
    c. the person experiencing the event is passive and inner-directed.
    d. the person experiencing the event is highly sensitive to criticism and suspicious of others.

14. What is a fear network?
    a. A memory network that interconnects the fear stimuli and response elements associated with severe trauma.
    b. A PTSD prevention team which is usually the first on the scene to deal with a victim's trauma.
    c. A PTSD social support network of persons who have had similar experiences.
    d. Different life events which are similar to the one which caused PTSD symptoms.

15. Posttraumatic stress disorder
   a.   is not treatable.
   b.   can be effectively treated with drug therapy alone.
   c.   rarely involves the use of exposure to feared stimuli because it is too painful for the person to relive the experience.
   d.   commonly includes either imaginal or in vivo exposure in conjunction with other cognitive techniques as well as medication.

Answers to test your understanding

1. a.   (7-10)
2. b.   (7-10)
3. d.   (7-10)
4. c.   (7-11)
5. a.   (7-12)
6. d.   (7-13)
7. a.   (7-13)
8. b.   (7-14)
9. b. d. (7-14)
10. c.   (7-15)
11. d.   (7-16)
12. b.   (7-16)
13. b.   (7-17)
14. a.   (7-17)
15. d.   (7-18)

When you have finished . . .

Explore the Web to find more information

If you're looking for information on the anxiety disorders a good place to start is **The National Institutes of Mental Health's Anxiety Disorders Information Page**. You will find material on specific disorders there, as well as an excellent link titled, How to Get Help for Anxiety Disorder and other links for more information. The URL is (**http://www.nimh.nih.gov/publicat/anxiety.htm**).

The National Institutes of Mental Health also provides an in depth body of information on obsessive-compulsive disorder at (**http://www.mentalhealth.com/book/p45-ocd1.html**). Some of the links provided are:

What is OCD?
How common is OCD?
Key Features of OCD
What causes OCD?
Do I have OCD?
Treatment of OCD: Progress Through Research
How to Get Help for OCD
What the Family Can Do to Help
If You Have Special Needs
For Further Information
References

More information about Tourette's disorder (previous to the publication of the DSM-IV it was called Tourette Syndrome), which is closely related to OCD, is available through the **National Tourette Syndrome Association**, (**http://neuro-www2.mgh.harvard.edu/tsa/tsamain.nclk**), **The Tourette Syndrome Home Page**, (**http://www.umd.umich.edu/~infinit/tourette.html**) and the "Tourette Syndrome Primer," an excellent article provided by **Children and Adults with Attention Deficit Disorders** (**http://www.chadd.org/tsprime.htm**).

You can access articles about panic disorder from the **National Institutes of Mental Health** at the URLs below.

- "Panic Disorder" (**http://www.nimh.nih.gov/publicat/panfly.htm**)

- "Understanding Panic Disorder" (**http://www.nimh.nih.gov/publicat/upd.htm**)

- "Getting Treatment for Panic Disorder" (**http://www.nimh.nih.gov/publicat/gettreat.htm**)

- "Panic Disorder Treatment and Referral" (**http://www.nimh.nih.gov/publicat/pandtr.htm**)

If you are searching for material on posttraumatic stress disorder, the **National Center for PTSD** is a good place to start. Among many other resources, they offer **PILOTS** database Web interface which provides both a menu-like way to do simple searches and a command-driven "expert search" capability. You will also find a description and sample questions for the child and adolescent version of the **Clinician-Administered PTSD Scale (CAPS-CA)**. Instructions for obtaining the CAPS-CA are also given. The Center also provide **National Center Fact Sheets** which offer information on selected aspects of PTSD prepared for nonprofessional readers. All of this information is available at (**http://www.dartmouth.edu/dms/ptsd/**).

The Posttraumatic Stress Resources Page is another good place to start your search for information about PTSD. It is sponsored by the **Carl T. Hayden Veterans Affairs Medical Center** which is located at (**http://www.long-beach.va.gov/ptsd/stress.html**).

CHAPTER 8
Dissociative and Somatoform Disorders

Before you read . . .

Survey the chapter

Chapter 8 begins with the case of Louise, a thirty-year-old woman who is struggling with a number of problems, among them chronic physical complaints for which she can find no medical explanation or relief, as well as difficulties with her memory and dramatic alterations in her behavior. As you learn more about Louise, you will see that many of her problems fit into the two categories of mental disorder covered in this chapter, dissociative disorders and somatoform disorders.

Dissociative disorders involve disruptions in a person's memory, consciousness or identity. The dissociative disorders that are discussed in this chapter are dissociative identity disorder, which used to be called multiple personality disorder, dissociative amnesia, dissociative fugue and depersonalization disorder.

The other category of mental disorder covered in Chapter 8 is the somatoform disorders. These disorders describe a pattern of chronic physical complaints or disabilities that suggest a medical problem, but have no known biological cause. These disorders include somatization disorder, hypochondriasis, conversion disorder, pain disorder and body dysmorphic disorder. As you read this section of the chapter, remember that the complaints of persons suffering from these disorders should not be simply dismissed with the statement, "It's just in their heads." Their pain, discomfort and concern are real to the patient and the effects of somatoform disorders can be dramatically disabling.

As you read . . .

Ask questions

8-1   How did the concepts of dissociation and somatization develop?

8-2   What are the symptoms of dissociation? Is mild dissociation common? Is it seen in other cultures?

8-3   What is dissociative identity disorder (DID)?

8-4   Is dissociative identity disorder a real clinical disorder?

8-5   What is dissociative amnesia?

8-6   What is dissociative fugue?

8-7   What is depersonalization disorder?

8-8   Are some people more vulnerable to dissociative disorders than others?

8-9   What factors can cause dissociative identity disorder?

8-10   How is dissociative identity disorder treated?

8-11   How are other dissociative disorders treated?

8-12   What are the somatoform disorders?

8-13   What is somatization disorder?

8-14   What is hypochondriasis?

8-15   What is conversion disorder?

8-16   What is pain disorder?

8-17   What is body dysmorphic disorder?

8-18   What factors can cause the development of somatization disorders?

8-19   How are somatization disorders treated?

After you read . . .

Review and explore the chapter

8-1   How did the concepts of dissociation and somatization develop?

1.   Match the following.

     1.   ____ somatic
     2.   ____ hysteria
     3.   ____ conversion hysteria

4. ____ repression
5. ____ neurosis
6. ____ dissociation
7. ____ somatization

    a. the original classification for somatoform and dissociative disorders in the DSM-II

    b. from Greek word for uterus, it originally referred to a condition where a person had multiple somatic complaints without obvious medical explanation

    c. physical

    d. Freud's concept for unconsciously forgetting personally threatening material

    e. process in which the normally integrated processes of consciousness, memory and personal identity become splintered

    f. process in which physical symptoms which suggest a medical disorder appear without adequate medical explanation

    g. nineteenth century Freudian term describing a condition where overwhelming anxiety had been converted into a physical symptom

---

8-2   What are the symptoms of dissociation? Is mild dissociation common? Is it seen in other cultures?

---

2. Dissociative experiences are not necessarily _____ (normal / pathological). In fact, mild forms of dissociation are _____ (symptomatic of mental disorder / common and perfectly normal).

3. a. What are some examples of common dissociation?

    b. When does dissociation become symptomatic of mental disorder?

4. Is mild dissociation common in other cultures? In your own words, provide a few examples.

5.   Fill in the missing information in the table below.

KEY SYMPTOMS OF MOST DISSOCIATIVE DISORDERS	DESCRIPTION OF KEY SYMPTOMS
Amnesia	
Depersonalization	
Derealization	
	an uncertainty about the nature of a person's own identity, of who he or she is
Identity Alteration	

8-3	What is dissociative identity disorder (DID)?

6.   Dissociative identity disorder (DID) was known as _____ (multiple personality disorder / schizophrenia) prior to the DSM-IV. Once thought to be an extremely _____ (common / uncommon) disorder, the number of reported cases in North America has dramatically _____ (decreased / increased) in the last two decades. In dissociative identity disorder, an individual's personality appears as _____ (separate / nonexistent) identities, rather than an integrated cohesive whole. DID is diagnosed much more often in _____ (women / men), and most cases are thought to be the result of _____ (genetic inheritance / childhood trauma such as extreme abuse).

7.   Match the following.

1.   ____ alters
2.   ____ host personality
3.   ____ personality fragments
4.   ____ switching

    a.   less well-developed than alters, typically represent one emotion such as rage

    b.   individual personalities

    c.   the primary identity in charge most of the time

    d.   the process of changing from one personality to another

| 8-4 | Is dissociative identity disorder a real clinical disorder? |

8. a. Some mental health professionals doubt that dissociative identity disorder is a true separate mental disorder. In your own words, describe three of their arguments.

1.

2.

3.

b. In your own words, discuss the common argument often used by those who believe that DID is a true mental disorder.

| 8-5 | What is dissociative amnesia? |

9. What is the key symptom of dissociative amnesia?

10. Match the following.

1. ____ localized amnesia
2. ____ selective amnesia
3. ____ generalized amnesia
4. ____ continuous amnesia
5. ____ systematized amnesia

a. total loss of memory of a person's entire life

b. loss of memory of events from a particular time or trauma up to the present

c.   loss of memory of a distinct period of time, usually a few hours, immediately after a trauma

d.   the loss of memory of certain classes of information

e.   loss of memory of some events surrounding a trauma

8-6   What is dissociative fugue?

11. a.   What are the major features of dissociative fugue?

b.   How long do most fugue states last?

c.   What kinds of events precipitate fugue states?

d.   How do most persons in fugue states behave?

8-7   What is depersonalization disorder?

12. a.   In your own words, briefly describe depersonalization disorder.

b.   Why is it important to rule out other mental and physical problems when making a diagnosis of depersonalization disorder?

| 8-8 | Are some people more vulnerable to dissociative disorders than others? |

13. In your own words, briefly describe the following factors which seem to relate to a person's tendency to dissociate.

    a.   imaginative involvement

    b.   hypnotizability

    c.   childhood trauma

| 8-9 | What factors can cause dissociative identity disorder? |

14. In your own words, briefly describe and discuss the two major theories which attempt to explain the development of dissociative identity disorder.

    a.   trauma-dissociation model

       1.   description:

       2.   evaluation:

    b.   sociocultural model

       1.   description:

       2.   evaluation:

| 8-10 | How is dissociative identity disorder treated? |

15. a. Many therapists believe that if treatment of DID is to be successful, the alters have to be fused in therapy. What do they mean by that?

    b. In your own words, briefly describe each of the four phases of therapy often seen in long-term individual psychotherapy for DID.

        1. phase one

        2. phase two

        3. phase three

        4. phase four

| 8-11 | How are other dissociative disorders treated? |

16. Most individuals with dissociative amnesia, fugue or depersonalization disorder improve _____ (without formal treatment / only with intensive therapy), once the _____ (triggering stressor / brain chemistry imbalance) has been removed or resolved.

17. Why has the development of specific treatments for depersonalization and derealization symptoms received so little attention?

Test your understanding

1. The process in which the normally integrated processes of consciousness, memory and personal identity become splintered is called
   a. repression.
   b. dissociation.
   c. somatization.
   d. neurosis.

2. The process in which physical symptoms which suggest a medical disorder appear without adequate medical explanation
   a. is called repression.
   b. is called dissociation.
   c. is called somatization.
   d. is called neurosis.

3. In the DSM-II, somatoform and dissociative disorders were categorized as a type of
   a. repression.
   b. dissociation.
   c. somatization.
   d. neurosis.

4. The process of dissociation
   a. is always a sign of pathology.
   b. is seen only in North America and Western Europe.
   c. becomes symptomatic of mental disorder when it is distressing and impairs functioning.
   d. occurs only in dissociative disorders.

5. The process of depersonalization describes
   a. persistent feelings of detachment, including out-of-body experiences and control.
   b. significant memory loss.
   c. behavioral patterns which suggest that the person has assumed a new sense of identity.
   d. a sense that the external world has somehow become strange or unreal.

6. Dissociative identity disorder
   a. is a subtype of schizophrenia.
   b. is diagnosed more often in men than in women.
   c. is diagnosed more often today than it was twenty years ago.
   d. is always caused by genetic inheritance.

7. Mental health professionals who view dissociative identity disorder as a true separate mental disorder, respond to critics by pointing out that
   a. DID is not a cultural bound syndrome seen mainly in North America and Western Europe.
   b. the symptoms of DID do not overlap into other disorders.
   c. the features of DID are almost impossible to create through suggestion.
   d. it would be extremely difficult for a person to successfully mimic or fake many of the physical and behavioral symptoms of DID.

8. Localized amnesia refers to a
   a. total loss of memory of a person's life.
   b. loss of memory of events from a particular time or trauma up to the present.
   c. loss of memory of a distinct period of time, usually a few hours, immediately after a trauma.
   d. loss of memory of some events surrounding a trauma.

9. Generalized amnesia refers to a
   a. total loss of memory of a person's life.
   b. loss of memory of events from a particular time or trauma up to the present.
   c. loss of memory of a distinct period of time, usually a few hours, immediately

after a trauma.

d.   loss of memory of some events surrounding a trauma.

10. Which of the following statements about dissociative fugue is not true?
    a.   A central feature of fugue is traveling.
    b.   Most fugue states last only a few days, but they can go on for months.
    c.   Most fugue states are precipitated by traumatic events or overwhelming everyday stressors.
    d.   Persons in fugue states act in very strange and peculiar ways.

11. Which of the following statements about depersonalization disorder is not true?
    a.   A central feature of depersonalization disorder are distressing dreamlike feelings of depersonalization.
    b.   A central feature of depersonalization disorder is distressing dreamlike feelings of derealization.
    c.   Depersonalization and derealization experiences are rare and always indicate depersonalization disorder whether the person is distressed or not.
    d.   It is important to rule out other mental and physical problems before making a diagnosis of depersonalization disorder.

12. Which of the following factors tend to increase a person's tendency to dissociate?
    a.   traumatic abuse during childhood
    b.   difficultly engaging in imaginative involvement
    c.   lack of response to hypnotic suggestion, especially in adulthood
    d.   such high levels of social support that it becomes overwhelming

13. The sociocultural model of the development of dissociative identity disorder
    a.   emphasizes the role of childhood abuse.
    b.   emphasizes the role of drug abuse.
    c.   emphasizes the idea that DID is a social role often learned from the

therapist.

d.   Emphasizes the fact that DID is diagnosed mainly in white, middle-to-upper class females.

14. Many therapists believe that if treatment for dissociative identity disorder is to be successful, the alters must be
    a.   ignored.
    b.   fused.
    c.   further fragmented.
    d.   brought to an agreement as to which alter performs which social role.

15. Most persons with dissociative amnesia, fugue or depersonalization disorder
    a.   never recover.
    b.   improve without formal treatment.
    c.   improve, but only with intensive therapy.
    d.   don't need therapy, because the vast majority of them are faking.

Answers to test your understanding

1.	b.	(8-1)
2.	c.	(8-1)
3.	d.	(8-1)
4.	c.	(8-2)
5.	a.	(8-2)
6.	c.	(8-3)
7.	d.	(8-4)
8.	c.	(8-5)
9.	a.	(8-5)
10.	d.	(8-6)
11.	c.	(8-7)
12.	a.	(8-8)
13.	c.	(8-9)
14.	b.	(8-10)
15.	b.	(8-11)

| 8-12 | What are the somatoform disorders? |

18. Mark each of the following situations YES, if it fits your text's description of somatoform disorder and NO, if it does not.

a   ____   Seth falls out of a tree and breaks his leg.

b.   ____   After seeing an automobile accident, Ann suddenly becomes blind, even though no biological explanation can be found.

c.   ____   After slipping and falling, Andrew pretends to have back pain and sues the store owner.

d.   ____   Even though she has had three CAT scans that found nothing, every time Rebecca has a headache she worries for days that it might be a brain tumor.

19. What is meant by the term somatization?

20. a.   What is factitious disorder?

b.   Is factitious disorder the same thing as malingering? Why?

c.   How are somatoform disorders different from factitious disorder and malingering?

21. Why are somatoform disorders so difficult to diagnose?

| 8-13 | What is somatization disorder? |

22. In your own words, describe somatization disorder.

23. How does somatization disorder differ from undifferentiated somatoform disorder?

8-14	What is hypochondriasis?

24. In your own words, describe hypochondriasis.

25. In what ways are somatization disorder and hypochondriasis different?

8-15	What is conversion disorder?

26. In your own words, describe conversion disorder.

27. What are the three common types of symptoms seen in conversion disorder?

   a.

   b.

   c.

28. a.   What is la belle indifference?

b.   How can la belle indifference be used to differentiate between true conversion disorder and malingering?

8-16   What is pain disorder?

---

29. In your own words, describe pain disorder.

30. What is the difference between acute pain disorder and chronic pain disorder?

8-17   What is body dysmorphic disorder?

---

31. In your own words, describe body dysmorphic disorder.

32. How does body dysmorphic disorder differ from normal concern about one's physical appearance or common vanity?

8-18   What factors can cause the development of somatization disorders?

---

33. The diathesis-stress model, which is used to describe how somatoform disorders are caused, is based on three elements. Describe them below in your own words.

a.

b.

c.

34. In your own words, briefly describe how each of the following concepts are tied to biological or psychological vulnerabilities to develop various somatoform disorders.

   a.   impulsive behavior

   b.   the right hemisphere of the brain

   c.   somatosensory amplifiers

   d.   private self-consciousness

   e.   negative affectivity

   f.   family attitudes

   g.   recurrent abdominal pain

35. In your own words, briefly describe the role of childhood stress and trauma in the development of various somatoform disorders.

36. In your own words, briefly describe the role of secondary gain in the development of various somatoform disorders.

8-19	How are somatization disorders treated?

37. Fill in the missing information in the table below.

SOMATOFORM DISORDER	TYPICAL TREATMENT(S)
Somatization Disorder and Hypochondriasis	
Conversion Disorder	
Body Dysmorphic Disorder	
Pain Disorder	

Test your understanding

1. Somatoform disorders
   a. involve physical complaints or disabilities for which no organic cause can be found.
   b. involve situations where a person exaggerates or pretends to have symptoms.
   c. involve situations where a person pretends to have symptoms in order to avoid something.
   d. are not true mental disorders.

2. Harriet has visited a variety of doctors over the last six years seeking relief from many different physical complaints. No underlying physical explanation for any of her symptoms has ever been found. Harriet's problems are consistent with
   a. hypochondriasis.
   b. somatization disorder.
   c. la belle indifference.
   d. dissociation.

3. Why are somatization disorders so hard to diagnose?
   a. Because the patient consciously tries to avoid discovery that his or her symptoms are fake.
   b. Because the patient unconsciously tries to avoid discovery that his or her symptoms are fake.
   c. Because symptoms tend to mimic physical disorders, physicians often have difficulty determining the underlying cause.
   d. Because people with somatization disorder rarely seek medical treatment.

4. In order to make a diagnosis of somatization disorder
    a. the pattern of physical complaints must last for no longer than three weeks.
    b. the person must have had fewer than four different physical complaints.
    c. the complaints must have been serious enough to warrant the desire for medical treatment or have interfered with daily functioning.
    d. an underlying physical explanation must be found for at least 80 percent of the complaints.

5. If a person presents fewer than eight somatic complaints which have lasted for at least six months and are not caused by a medical condition, the correct diagnosis would be
    a. somatization disorder.
    b. undifferentiated somatoform disorder.
    c. uncommon somatization disorder.
    d. somatoform disorder of unknown type.

6. After walking up three flights of stairs, Bob notices that his pulse rate has increased and soon he is in turmoil worrying that this may indicate that he has heart trouble. He goes to the doctor for reassurance. Bob's actions are consistent with
    a. hypochondriasis.
    b. somatization disorder.
    c. la belle indifference.
    d. possible heart disease.

7. After viewing an automobile accident, Ann suddenly goes blind. No underlying neurological explanation for her blindness can be found. Ann's behavior is consistent with
    a. hypochondriasis.
    b. somatization disorder.
    c. conversion disorder.
    d. la belle indifference.

8. In a conversion disordered patient, a seemingly indifferent and nonchalant attitude toward his or her loss of function is

commonly seen. This is called
    a. hypochondriasis.
    b. malingering.
    c. factitious behavior.
    d. la belle indifference.

9. Acute pain disorder describes
    a. complaints of pain, thought to have psychological causes, which last for less than six months.
    b. complaints of pain, thought to have psychological causes, which last for more than six months.
    c. an inability to perceive pain which lasts for less than six months.
    d. an inability to perceive pain which lasts for more than six months.

10. Ted has body dysmorphic disorder. This means that
    a. Ted is an unattractive person.
    b. Ted suffers from tremendous anxiety because he is unattractive.
    c. Ted is a normal looking person who is concerned with his appearance.
    d. Ted is a normal looking person who perceives himself as ugly. He is so preoccupied with this concern, that he stays in his house for days in order to avoid going out into public.

11. The diathesis-stress model, which is used to describe how somatoform disorders are caused, is based on three elements. Which of the following is not one of these elements?
    a. A predisposition to somatoform disorders is conveyed by a combination of biological and psychological vulnerabilities.
    b. Biological and psychological vulnerabilities interact with stressors from the environment to cause physical arousal.
    c. Symptoms of physical arousal are interpreted by the person as signs of physical illness.

d. The person recognizes the perceived symptoms as unrelated to their actual physical health.

12. Somatosensory amplifiers
   a. are located on the right side of the brain.
   b. describe an enhanced perception of normal bodily sensations.
   c. describe problematic modeling, which occurs in families where illness is valued as a way to avoid responsibility.
   d. are related to the development of all of the somatoform disorders, except hypochondriasis.

13. The personality trait of negative affectivity describes
   a. a love of illness.
   b. the need to avoid responsibility by pretending to be sick.
   c. the tendency to worry, be pessimistic, fear uncertainty, feel guilt, tire easily and have poor self-esteem.
   d. the tendency to misperceive normal bodily sensations as symptoms of serious illness.

14. Do some researchers believe that childhood stress and traumatic abuse may play a role in the development of some somatoform disorders?
   a. No, because research clearly shows that there is no relationship between childhood abuse and later somatoform disorders.
   b. Yes, because childhood abuse can cause damage to the left side of the brain, increasing the chance of developing conversion disorder.
   c. Yes, because dissociation is usually the first step in the process of somatization.
   d. Yes, because young children can not express themselves verbally, they may learn to use illness as a way to express emotional distress.

15. Assigning a special case manager to help the patient reduce doctor shopping and constant help seeking is a common practice in the treatment of
   a. all somatoform disorders.
   b. somatization disorder and hypochondriasis.
   c. conversion disorder and body dysmorphic disorder.
   d. body dysmorphic disorder and pain disorder.

Answers to test your understanding

1.	a.	(8-12)
2.	b.	(8-12)
3.	c.	(8-12)
4.	c.	(8-13)
5.	b.	(8-13)
6.	a.	(8-14)
7.	c.	(8-15)
8.	d.	(8-15)
9.	a.	(8-16)
10.	c.	(8-17)
11.	d.	(8-18)
12.	b.	(8-18)
13.	c.	(8-18)
14.	d.	(8-18)
15.	b.	(8-19)

When you have finished . . .

Explore the Web to find more information

The International Society for the Study of Dissociation home page offers a short list of links to other sites. You may also find their link <u>Guidelines for Treating Dissociative Identity Disorder In Adults</u> interesting. (**http://www.issd.org/**).

A very interesting Web site which is devoted to providing information and support for MPD/DID is **DividedHearts**. You can locate them at (**http://www.netdesigns2000.com/mpd/**).

The Psychiatric Institute of Washington provides the article, "The Spectrum of Dissociative Disorders: An Overview of Diagnosis and Treatment," by Joan A. Turkus, M.D., as well as a bibliography of books, magazines and journals which deal with abuse, trauma and dissociative disorders. You can find this page at (**http://www.voiceofwomen.com/center.html**).

Internet Mental Health provides the article, "First Aid for Somatizers," The Harvard Mental Health Letter, August, 1995, at (**http://www.mentalhealth.com/mag1/p5h-sm01.html**).

CHAPTER 9
Mood Disorders and Suicide

Before you read . . .

Survey the chapter

Chapter 9 begins with the case of Margaret, and her slow descent into the black hole of depression. As you read about Margaret, notice that the symptoms of her depression are more than simply an extension of negative emotional feelings that we all encounter from time to time. Clinical depression involves a complex cluster of problems, stealing pleasure from our lives, affecting how we view ourselves and our loved ones, how we sleep, eat, move and even process our own thoughts.

This chapter considers the mood disorders in detail, examining their symptoms and patterns, causes and the efforts of mental health professionals to design effective methods for prevention and treatment. Chapter 9 concludes with a discussion of the most devastating behavior sometimes associated with depression, suicide.

As you read . . .

Ask questions

9-1   What is meant by the concept of mood disorder?

9-2   At what point does depression become serious enough to qualify as a mental disorder?

9-3   What are the typical features of major depressive disorder?

9-4   What is the typical course of major depression?

9-5   Are there subtypes of major depressive disorder?

9-6   What is dysthymic disorder? Are there other types of depression?

9-7   What are the features of bipolar disorder?

9-8   How are bipolar disorders classified?

9-9   What is cyclothymic disorder?

9-10   Can genetic factors influence the development of mood disorders?

9-11   Can neurobiological dysfunction influence the development of mood disorders?

9-12   Can depression be related to problems with intimate relationships?

9-13   Can depression be learned or influenced by cognitive processes in other ways?

9-14   How can stressors trigger depressive episodes?

9-15   Is there a relationship between personality traits, coping skills and depression?

9-16   How are medications used in the treatment of mood disorders?

9-17   How are electroconvulsive therapy and light therapy used to treat mood disorders?

9-18   What kinds of psychologically-based therapies are used to treat mood disorders?

9-19   Are biologically-based and psychologically-based therapies for mood disorders more effective if they are combined?

9-20   Who is at greatest risk for attempting and completing suicide?

9-21   What causal factors are associated with suicide?

After you read . . .

Review and explore the chapter

9-1   What is meant by the concept of mood disorder?

1.   The concept of mood disorder refers to a _____ (specific emotional disturbance / group of emotional disturbances) associated with serious and persistent difficulty maintaining _____ (happiness / an even and productive emotional state). Mood disorders are also referred to by clinicians as _____ (affective disorders / nervous breakdowns). The most common mood disorder in Western culture is _____ (mania / depression).

2. Mood disorders, such as depression, involve more than just emotional symptoms. In what other ways can they affect a person's life?

3. Are mood disorders and creativity linked? If so, how?

9-2   At what point does depression become serious enough to qualify as a mental disorder?

---

4. Everyone goes through periods of time when they are sad or blue. What are three characteristics that differentiate those experiences from a depressive disorder?

    a.

    b.

    c.

5. It is estimated that one in _____ (five / twenty-five) adults in the United States will experience at least one episode of significant depression at some time in their life. Females are _____ (not / twice) as likely to experience significant depression. Depressive disorders _____ (are / are not) related to a specific socioeconomic status and can occur _____ (at any age / only in adulthood).

6. a. What are common problems which are often comorbid with depression?

    b. What is meant by negative affect?

9-3	What are the typical features of major depressive disorder?

7. Using the table below, describe some of the common characteristics of major depressive episodes.

BEHAVIORAL AREA		TYPICAL SYMPTOMS OF DEPRESSIVE EPISODES
Mood Symptoms (most common)	What is the effect on mood?	There is despair and constant sadness. For example, the person feels that she is in a deep black hole, that she is totally worthless and that the situation is hopeless.
	How does the person view his or her life?	There is a loss of the ability to enjoy activities central to a person's life (anhedonia). For example, an avid fisherman, no longer finds fishing enjoyable.
Physical Symptoms	What is the effect on appetite?	
	What is the effect on energy level and movement?	
	What is the effect on somatic complaints?	
	What is the effect on sleep?	
	What is the effect on the immune system?	
Cognitive Symptoms	What is the effect on self-esteem?	
	Is concentration affected?	
	Who does the person blame for his or her problems?	
	How does the person view the future and past?	

8. a. What psychotic symptoms are sometimes seen in the most severe cases of major depression?

    b. What is meant when psychotic symptoms which are comorbid with major depression are termed mood congruent?

9. Why is it important for family practice and primary care physicians to be not only aware of depression, but also to be careful before a diagnosis of depression is made?

9-4   What is the typical course of major depression?

---

10. Most cases of major depressive episodes clear up, even without treatment, in a matter of _____ (days / months). In some cases, adults who experience one episode of major depression fully recover and never have another episode. More commonly, however, in perhaps as many as _____ (one quarter / three-quarters) of cases, episodes of major depression are recurrent, with studies finding that depressed patients suffer an average of _____ (five to six / one hundred to two hundred) episodes in their lifetimes. Although major depressive disorder can begin at any age, the most typical age of first onset is in the middle _____ (twenties / forties).

11. What is double depression?

9-5   Are there subtypes of major depressive disorder?

---

12. Match the following DSM-IV specifiers to the correct definition.

    1. ____ chronic
    2. ____ with atypical features
    3. ____ with melancholic features
    4. ____ with catatonic features
    5. ____ with seasonal pattern
    6. ____ with postpartum onset

    a. This specifier would be used for a case that begins within four weeks after the birth of a child.

b.   This specifier would be used in the case of a person who becomes depressed only during the winter months.

c.   This specifier would be used in a case that includes severe anhedonia (being unable to get back to sleep after awaking early), extreme agitation or slowness and/or significant weight loss.

d.   This specifier would be used in a case where symptoms of major depressive disorder have lasted for more than two years.

e.   This specifier would be used in a case where the depression is marked with extreme psychomotor (movement) disturbances.

f.   This specifier is applied to a case where the symptoms do not follow the usual patterns of major depressive disorder.

9-6   What is dysthymic disorder? Are there other types of depression?

13. In your own words, briefly describe the typical characteristics of dysthymic disorder.

14. In what circumstance would a clinician use the following diagnostic categories?

a.   adjustment disorder

b.   bereavement

9-7   What are the features of bipolar disorder?

15. Bipolar disorder, which is also called _____ (mixed mood / manic-depressive) disorder, includes periods of depression as well as periods of mania, which is _____ (a lack of / an extremely elevated) mood, or mixed episodes in which episodes of depression and mania alternate _____ (rapidly, within the same day / slowly, taking months to complete a cycle).

16. Although major depressive disorder and bipolar disorder overlap in many ways, they are also quite different. In your own words, briefly describe five major differences between major depressive

disorder and bipolar disorder.

a.

b.

c.

d.

e.

17. Using the table below, describe some of the common characteristics of manic episodes.

	TYPICAL SYMPTOMS OF MANIC EPISODES
What is the effect on mood?	
What is the effect on sleep?	
What is the effect on speech?	
What is the effect on judgement?	
What is the effect on thought processing?	
What is the effect on concentration?	

What is the effect on sense of self-esteem?	

18. In your own words, briefly discuss the similarities and differences between mania, hyperactivity and psychosis.

9-8	How are bipolar disorders classified?

19. Match the following.

1. ____ bipolar I disorder
2. ____ bipolar II disorder
3. ____ hypomanic
4. ____ with rapid cycling
5. ____ with/without full interepisode recovery

    a.   specifier is used when four or more mood episodes are experienced within one year

    b.   used when hypomanic episodes are interspersed with depression

    c.   used when full-blown mania is interspersed with depression

    d.   term used to describe relatively mild manic episodes

    e.   specifier which describes mood between episodes of mania and depression

9-9	What is cyclothymic disorder?

20. In your own words, briefly describe the typical characteristics of cyclothymic disorder.

Test your understanding

1.   The most common mood disorder in Western culture is
     a.   depression.
     b.   mania.
     c.   manic depression.
     d.   dysthymic disorder.

2.   How do mood disorders such as major depression affect a person's life?
     a.   Mood disorders are mainly focused on problems with the person's self-concept.
     b.   Mood disorders are mainly focused on problems with the person's personal relationships.
     c.   Mood disorders are mainly focused on problems with the person's ability to work or go to school.
     d.   Mood disorders negatively affect almost all aspects of a person's life.

3.   Which of the following is not one of the major differences between clinical depression and the occasional sad mood we all experience from time to time?
     a.   The depression lasts much longer.
     b.   The depression impairs the person's ability to function.
     c.   The depression is always mixed with periods of extreme mania.
     d.   There is a cluster of other physical and behavioral symptoms associated with the negative mood.

4.   It is estimated that one in every _____ adults in the United States will experience at least one episode of significant depression at some point in their life.
     a.   five
     b.   twenty-five
     c.   fifty
     d.   seventy-five

5.   What are the two most common symptoms of major depressive disorder?
     a.   difficulty sleeping, loss of appetite
     b.   extreme despair, loss of pleasure and interest in life activities
     c.   crying, sleeping all the time
     d.   alcoholism, suicide

6.   Which of the following is not characteristic of a typical depressive episode?
     a.   lack of energy
     b.   difficulty concentrating
     c.   always blaming others for problems
     d.   increased complaints of bodily aches and pains

7.   Which of the following statements about major depressive episodes is true?
     a.   Most major depressive episodes clear up, even without treatment, in a matter of months.
     b.   Fewer than one percent of adults who experience one episode of major depression fully recover and never have another episode.
     c.   Studies find that patients who suffer from recurrent episodes of depression average between one hundred and two hundred episodes in their lifetimes.
     d.   Although major depressive disorder can begin at any age, the most typical age of first onset is in the middle forties.

8.   Bob's symptoms of major depression occur only during the winter months. His diagnosis would be
     a.   major depressive disorder with atypical features.
     b.   major depressive disorder with melancholiac features.
     c.   major depressive disorder with winter onset.
     d.   major depressive disorder with seasonal pattern.

9. Which disorder describes a chronic ongoing depressive state which is disruptive, though less disabling to a person's life than major depressive disorder, and lasts at least two years?
   a. major depressive disorder with atypical features
   b. dysthymic disorder
   c. cyclothymic disorder
   d. double depression

10. Bipolar disorder
    a. includes periods of mania with no depressive episodes.
    b. includes periods of depression simultaneously occurring with hyperactivity.
    c. is also called manic-depression.
    d. in most cases reaches psychotic levels.

11. Which of the following is not one of the major differences between major depressive disorder and bipolar disorder?
    a. Major depressive disorder is more common in women, while men and women are at equal risk for bipolar disorder.
    b. Bipolar disorder usually begins in the late teens or early twenties, which is earlier than major depressive disorder.
    c. Bipolar disorder seems to occur more frequently among higher socioeconomic status groups.
    d. Bipolar disorder probably has no genetic basis, while major depressive disorder is almost always tied to genetic factors.

12. Which of the following is a typical symptom of manic episodes?
    a. engaging in ill-advised, dangerous or promiscuous behaviors
    b. increased concentration, which is due to the person's racing thoughts
    c. the ability to fall asleep almost anywhere at anytime
    d. lowered self-esteem

13. A person is presenting full-blown episodes of mania interspersed with periods of depression. The most accurate diagnosis would be
    a. cyclothymic disorder.
    b. bipolar I disorder.
    c. bipolar II disorder.
    d. bipolar III disorder.

14. The term hypomanic is used to describe
    a. manic and depressive symptoms occurring at the same time.
    b. extreme and dramatic manic episodes.
    c. relatively mild manic episodes.
    d. a person who consistently worries that he or she may develop bipolar disorder.

15. A chronic fluctuation between depression and mania which is not severe enough to warrant a diagnosis of bipolar disorder is called
    a. dysthymic disorder.
    b. cyclothymic disorder.
    c. bipolar I disorder.
    d. double depression.

Answers to test your understanding

1.	a.	(9-1)
2.	d.	(9-1)
3.	c.	(9-2)
4.	a.	(9-2)
5.	b.	(9-3)
6.	c.	(9-3)
7.	a.	(9-4)
8.	d.	(9-5)
9.	b.	(9-6)
10.	c.	(9-7)
11.	d.	(9-7)
12.	a.	(9-7)
13.	b.	(9-8)
14.	c.	(9-8)
15.	b.	(9-9)

| 9-10 | Can genetic factors influence the development of mood disorders? |

21. a.   Taken together, twin, adoption and family studies suggest that genetic factors _____ (play / do not play) a role in mood disorders, but that their influence is stronger in _____ (unipolar / bipolar) than in _____ (unipolar / bipolar) depression. These studies also show that there is a much more clearly defined genetic risk for _____ (unipolar depression / bipolar disorder) than for _____ (dysthymia / cyclothymia).

    b.   Can genetics alone explain the causal factors of mood disorders? Why or why not?

| 9-11 | Can neurobiological dysfunction influence the development of mood disorders? |

22. a.   In your own words, briefly describe the original catecholamine theory of depression.

    b.   In your own words, briefly summarize the findings of recent research into the role of neurotransmitters and depression.

23.   Recent research has found that in some cases both depression and mania are accompanied by low levels of the neurotransmitter serotonin. What are two possible explanations for this paradox?

    a.

    b.

24.   In your own words, briefly describe the possible role of the hypothalamic-pituitary-adrenal axis in depression.

9-12	Can depression be related to problems with intimate relationships?

25. Summarize the following theories of interpersonal relationships and mood disorder in the table below.

THEORY	SUMMARY OF MAIN POINTS
Psychoanalytic Theory (Freud)	
Attachment Theory (Bowlby)	
Interpersonal Theories	

9-13	Can depression be learned or influenced by cognitive processes in other ways?

26. Summarize the following learning and cognition theories of mood disorder in the table below.

THEORY	SUMMARY OF MAIN POINTS
The Reinforcement Model (Lewinsohn)	
The Self-control Model (Rehm)	
Learned Helplessness	
Cognitive Theory (Beck)	
Self-awareness Theory (Pyszczynski and Greenberg)	

9-14	How can stressors trigger depressive episodes?

27. a.   Your text states that many theorists view depression from a diathesis-stress perspective. What is meant by this?

b.   What are some examples of environmental events which may be closely linked to depression?

| 9-15 | Is there a relationship between personality traits, coping skills and depression? |

28. a.   Some people tend to cope with stressors by using distraction. What does this mean?

b.   Is the use of distraction an effective coping mechanism in avoiding problems with depression? Why?

29. a.   Some people tend to cope with stressors by using rumination. What does this mean?

b.   Is the use of rumination an effective coping mechanism in avoiding problems with depression? Why?

30. a.   What are the traits of dependent (sociotropic) personality?

b.   Are people with dependent personality traits more susceptible to depression? Why?

31. a.   What are the traits of achievement (autonomy-oriented) personality?

b.   Are people with achievement personality traits more susceptible to depression? Why?

9-16   How are medications used in the treatment of mood disorders?

32. Fill in the missing information in the table below.

ANTIDEPRESSANT CATEGORY	TRADE NAMES	PHYSIOLOGICAL EFFECT(S)
Monoamine Oxidase (MAO) inhibitors	Nardil Parnate	
Tricyclics		
Selective Serotonin Reuptake Inhibitors (SSRIs)		
	Wellbutrin	

33. a.   What is lithium carbonate?

    b.   Why must persons taking lithium be closely monitored?

    c.   What other drugs are often used to treat the symptoms of bipolar disorder?

9-17   How are electroconvulsive therapy and light therapy used to treat mood disorders?

34. a.   What prompted the development of electroconvulsive therapy (ECT) more than sixty years ago?

    b.   How is ECT performed today in order to minimize problematic side effects?

c.   When is ECT most likely to be considered as a possible treatment?

35. In your own words, describe the use of light therapy in the treatment of mood disorder. Include the kind of mood disorder light therapy is used for and how this approach is administered.

9-18   What kinds of psychologically-based therapies are used to treat mood disorders?

---

36. In your own words, briefly describe each of the following psychologically-based treatments for mood disorders.

a.   psychodynamic approaches

b.   behavioral approaches

c.   cognitive-behavioral therapy

d.   interpersonal therapy

9-19   Are biologically-based and psychologically-based therapies for mood disorders more effective if they are combined?

---

37. Is it clear from research that combining psychologically and biologically-based therapies is the most effective method for treating major depression?

38. In general, how is medication and psychotherapy combined to treat bipolar disorder?

| 9-20 | Who is at greatest risk for attempting and completing suicide? |

---

39. Approximately _____ (15 percent / 50 percent) of depressed individuals eventually commit suicide. In the general population of the United States, about one in _____ (eight / eight hundred) suicide attempts results in a completed suicide. The best predictor of a subsequent suicide is _____ (severe depression / a previous suicide attempt).

40. a.   Are attempted suicides higher among men or women? What about completed suicides?

     b.   Are attempted suicides higher among younger or older persons? What about completed suicides?

     c.   Completed suicides are highest among which ethnic group?

     d.   Which disorders are strongly associated with completed suicide?

41. a.   What is the risk/rescue ratio? What does a high risk/rescue ratio signify?

42. a.   There has been a dramatic _____ (increase / decrease) in suicide rates for adolescents in the United States in the last thirty years. Approximately _____ (2,000 / 50,000) U.S. teenagers commit suicide each year, with the largest increase occurring among _____ (White / Black / Hispanic) _____ (females / males).

b.   In your own words, briefly describe each of the following ways in which adolescent suicide differs from suicide of adults?

1.   precipitating stressor

2.   contagion effect

3.   suicide pacts

9-21   What causal factors are associated with suicide?

43.   At the present time, is there consensus among researchers as to the role of genetics and neurotransmitter abnormalities in suicide?

44.   a.   Social and cultural indulgences seem to be _____ (strongly related / unrelated) to the prevalence of suicide.

b.   Match the following.

1.   ____ egoistic suicides
2.   ____ altruistic suicides
3.   ____ anomic suicides
4.   ____ fatalistic suicides

a.   Luis commits suicide after losing his job of thirty-four years.

b.   Eighty-year-old Maria commits suicide due to extreme loneliness and isolation.

c.   Robert sees his plight as hopeless and commits suicide in his jail cell.

d.   Tasha's suicide was made to look like an automobile accident. She was motivated by the fact that her life insurance would help pay for her son's needed operation.

Test your understanding

1. Studies show that
   a. genetic factors do not play a role in mood disorders.
   b. genetic factors totally control both the development and course of both unipolar and bipolar mood disorders.
   c. genetic factors play a role in mood disorders, but their influence is stronger in unipolar than in bipolar depression.
   d. genetic factors play a role in mood disorders, but their influence is stronger in bipolar than in unipolar depression.

2. The original catecholamine theory of depression
   a. stated that low levels of norepinephrine lead to depression and high levels of norepinephrine lead to mania.
   b. stated that high levels of norepinephrine lead to depression and low levels of norepinephrine lead to mania.
   c. stated that low levels of serotonin and dopamine lead to depression and high levels of serotonin and dopamine lead to mania.
   d. stated that high levels of serotonin and dopamine lead to depression and low levels of serotonin and dopamine lead to mania.

3. Recent research into the role of neurotransmitters and depression has found all of the following to be true, except that
   a. neurotransmitters other than norepinephrine, such as serotonin and dopamine, are also involved.
   b. not only the amount, but also the interaction between neurotransmitters may be important.
   c. both short-term as well as long-term changes in neurotransmitter function may be at work.

   d. most cases of major depression can be linked to problems with neurotransmitter function, while most of the cases of bipolar disorder cannot.

4. Bowlby's attachment theory is based on the assumption that
   a. depression is the result of unresolved conflicts involving the loss of a childhood caregiver.
   b. children with insecure attachments to adults do not learn to recognize distress or seek social support.
   c. unsatisfactory relationship patterns with others as an adult increase the risk of depression.
   d. the chemical make-up of the neurotransmitters of a young child are unstable until the age of ten.

5. The belief that people become more vulnerable to depression when they use negative self-schemas and distorted thinking patterns best describes
   a. the catecholamine theory of depression.
   b. the concept of learned helplessness.
   c. Beck's cognitive theory of depression.
   d. Freud's psychoanalytic theory of depression.

6. Which statement below best describes the diathesis-stress model of depression?
   a. A diathesis such as genetic inheritance or problems caused by dysfunctional social relationships predispose the person to environmental triggers, which then combine and result in depression.
   b. Persons with low levels of norepinephrine are at risk for depression, because they have a harder time attaching themselves to others.
   c. Persons with high levels of norepinephrine are at risk for depression, because they have a harder

time attaching themselves to others.

d. Depression is caused by either biological or psychosocial factors, but never both together.

7. Is rumination generally an effective way of coping with stressors and avoiding depression?
   a. Yes, because it helps the person focus totally on the stressor and find solutions.
   b. Yes, because it helps the person avoid the ineffective coping mechanism of distraction.
   c. No, because rumination often enhances the negative effect of the stressor and increases the severity and length of resulting depression.
   d. No, because rumination only helps people deal with stress if they are already taking an antidepressant medication.

8. Which of the following is not a characteristic trait of dependent (sociotropic) personality?
   a. a heightened sensitivity to isolation
   b. fear of abandonment
   c. a strong need for love from others
   d. more likely to become depressed over work-related failures and loss of status

9. The category of antidepressant drugs which works by blocking the enzyme that breaks down norepinephrine and serotonin is
   a. catecholamine blocking agents.
   b. MAO inhibitors.
   c. tricyclics.
   d. specific serotonin reuptake inhibitors (SSRIs).

10. The most commonly used medication for the treatment of bipolar disorder is
    a. lithium carbonate.
    b. Prozac.
    c. Wellbutrin.
    d. Antipole.

11. Which one of the following statements about electroconvulsive therapy (ECT) is not true?
    a. Clinicians are not clear on the reasons why ECT works, but it appears that the seizure, not the shock, is responsible for therapeutic effects.
    b. ECT is often effective with patients who do not respond to antidepressant medication.
    c. In order to minimize problematic side effects, ECT is administered only on one side of the head and medication to relax muscles and control heart rate, as well as oxygen are given.
    d. Although ECT was at one time a controversial form of treatment, today, it enjoys the support of almost all clinicians as well as the general public.

12. A depressed person who begins a program of interpersonal therapy can expect
    a. to attempt to uncover and explore long held unconsciousness conflicts.
    b. to learn new ways of enhancing support systems and interpersonal skills.
    c. to learn ways to reinforce healthy behavior, while extinguishing unhealthy depressive ones.
    d. to learn to avoid problematic thinking and negative assumptions about herself.

13. Is it clear from research that combining psychologically and biologically-based therapies is the most effective method for treating major depression?
    a. Yes, research consistently shows that antidepressant medications dramatically enhance the effects of psychotherapy.
    b. Yes, research consistently shows that psychotherapy dramatically enhances the effects of antidepressant medications.
    c. No, research consistently shows that combining psychotherapy and antidepressant medications is no more

effective than either treatment provided alone.

    d.   No, research findings have been mixed on this controversial question.

14. There has been a dramatic increase in suicide rates for adolescents in the United States in the last thirty years, with the largest increase occurring among
    a.   White males.
    b.   Black females.
    c.   Hispanic males.
    d.   Hispanic females.

15. When people commit suicide because they place the group ahead of their own survival, it is termed
    a.   egoistic suicide.
    b.   altruistic suicide.
    c.   anomic suicide.
    d.   fatalistic suicide.

Answers to test your understanding

1.   d.   (9-10)
2.   a.   (9-11)
3.   d.   (9-11)
4.   b.   (9-12)
5.   c.   (9-13)
6.   a.   (9-14)
7.   c.   (9-15)
8.   d.   (9-15)
9.   b.   (9-16)
10. a.   (9-16)
11. d.   (9-17)
12. b.   (9-18)
13. d.   (9-19)
14. a.   (9-20)
15. b.   (9-21)

When you have finished . . .

Explore the Web to find more information

A good general index of information about depression can be found at the **Internet Depression Resources List** which was compiled and is maintained by Dennis Taylor, (**http://www.execpc.com/~corbeau/**). This comprehensive and well maintained index is divided into links to:
    the Full List
    Treatment
    Depression
    Bipolar
    Panic
    Suicide

Another good starting point is the **Depression/Awareness, Recognition and Treatment (D/ART)** page located at (**http://www.nimh.nih.gov/newdart/darthome.htm**). It is sponsored by the **National Institutes of Mental Health** (NIMH), and is self-described as, ". . . a collaboration between the government and community organizations to benefit the mental health of the American public."

The Stanley Center for the Innovative Treatment of Bipolar Disorder provides a collection of published material on mood disorders at (**http://www.wpic.pitt.edu/research/stanley/othrinfo.htm**).

The following are provided by **Internet Mental Health**:

- "What is Bipolar II Disorder?" The Harvard Mental Health Letter, March, 1996. (**http://www.mentalhealth.com/mag1/p5h-bp02.html**)

- "Depression Rx for Teens No Longer 'Hit or Miss'?" by Pauline Anderson, The Medical Post, February 20, 1996. (**http://www.mentalhealth.com/mag1/p5m-dp02.html**)

- "Can Adolescent Suicide Be Prevented?" The Harvard Medical School Mental Health Letter, November, 1989. (**http://www.mentalhealth.com/mag1/p5h-sui4.html**)

The Columbia Presbyterian Medical Center provides two documents which deal with screening for depression and suicide.

- "Screening for Depression," (**http://cait.cpmc.columbia.edu/texts/gcps/gcps049.html**)

- "Screening for Suicidal Intent," (**http://cait.cpmc.columbia.edu/texts/gcps/gcps050.html**)

The following are provided by the Internet Mental Health:

Abuse. *DSM-IV: Essentials.* The Internet Mental Health Initiative. 9 September. <http://www.mentalhealth.com/mag1/p5h.html.>

Depression Reference Center, *2014 George Mason University*, by Pauline Anderson. December 20, 2003. <http://www.mentalhealth.com/mhn/...3-q60.html.>

Van Atonsson, Suicide Survivors. *The First ... ... Street.* 1 ... ... 1 ... tober 1996. <http://www.mentalhealth...com/mag1/p5h.m1.html.>

The Columbia Pediatrics Medical Center ... ... with resources for depression and suicide.

Remembering Bronterson. <http://teil.comm.columbia.edu/texts/p-q-q40373.html.>

Remembering Suicidal attempt. <http://ir... ...epid...com/mag-chinese-remember.html.>

CHAPTER 10
Schizophrenia

Before you read . . .

Survey the chapter

    Chapter 10 discusses schizophrenia and other psychoses, conditions which are among the most devastating and debilitating of the mental disorders. So far, the disorders that you have read about have primarily been centered around one specific aspect of a person's life. As you will see, schizophrenia is a much more global disorder, disrupting all of the most basic psychological functions. It can destroy the way a person perceives the world around them, as well as his or her beliefs in what is real and not real. It also negatively affects emotions, thinking patterns, speech, movements and the person's ability to relate to others.

    Schizophrenia will be discussed, including how the concept has been defined over the last 200 years, how the DSM-IV describes it today and how it differs from other psychotic disorders. You will then read about the lives of those afflicted with schizophrenia, the biological and psychosocial factors that may contribute to the development of the disorder and finally, the most effective methods in use today to control the symptoms of schizophrenia.

As you read . . .

Ask questions

10-1   What do clinicians mean by the concepts of psychosis and schizophrenia?

10-2   How has the concept of schizophrenia changed over time?

10-3   What is meant by positive symptoms of schizophrenia? What are they?

10-4   What is meant by negative symptoms of schizophrenia? What are they?

10-5   What are some of the other psychotic disorders and how do they differ from schizophrenia?

10-6   What is the course of schizophrenia?

10-7   Which persons are most likely to develop schizophrenia?

10-8   How is schizophrenia divided into subtypes by the DSM-IV and other classification systems?

10-9   Is schizophrenia related to genetic factors?

10-10   Is schizophrenia related to early physical trauma?

10-11   How are the brains of those suffering from schizophrenia different in structure and function?

10-12   What is the role of biochemical processes in schizophrenia?

10-13   What has been learned from the study of those people who are at risk for developing schizophrenia?

10-14   How are social class and place of residence related to schizophrenia?

10-15   Is early family environment related to schizophrenia?

10-16   Can the manner in which families express emotion be related to schizophrenia?

10-17   What biologically-based treatments are used to help control the symptoms of schizophrenia?

10-18   What psychosocial treatments are used to help control the symptoms of schizophrenia?

After you read . . .

Review and explore the chapter

| 10-1   What do clinicians mean by the concepts of psychosis and schizophrenia? |

1. In general the term _____ (neurosis / psychosis) refers to a serious mental disorder in which the individual lacks an accurate perception or understanding of reality and has little insight into how his or her behavior appears to others. These disorders can include periods of _____ (delusions / hallucinations) which are sensory experiences that seem real, but are not based on any external stimulation. Another common symptom is the presence of _____ (delusions / hallucinations) which are false beliefs about reality that are so firmly held that no evidence or argument can convince that person to give them up.   A third common element involves thinking and behavior patterns which are so _____ (enhanced / disorganized)) that onlookers often perceive these persons as _____ (crazy or insane / intelligent and insightful).

2. Is schizophrenia the same thing as dissociative identity disorder (multiple personality)?

3. In the table below, describe the various effects of schizophrenia on each of the basic psychological functions listed.

PSYCHOLOGICAL FUNCTION	PATTERN OF DISRUPTION CAUSED BY SCHIZOPHRENIA
Attention	
Perception	
Thought	
Emotion	
Behavior	
Social Interaction	

10-2	How has the concept of schizophrenia changed over time?

4. Match the following.

1. ____ John Haslam and Philippe Pinel
2. ____ Benedict Morel
3. ____ Emil Kraepelin
4. ____ Eugen Bleuler
5. ____ Kurt Schneider

a. He coined the term schizophrenia and categorized the symptoms as either primary or secondary.

b. Less than 200 years ago they were the first physicians to document the classic symptoms of schizophrenia.

c. He was the first to group the symptoms of schizophrenia into a separate syndrome which he called demence precoce (dementia praecox).

d. He helped to reduce problems in the diagnoses of schizophrenia by outlining easy to observe, "first rank" symptoms.

    e.   He differentiated dementia praecox from other known psychoses and divided it into hebephrenia, catatonic, paranoia and simple.

5.   What were Bleuler's four A's?

    a.

    b.

    c.

    d.

6.   According to the DSM-IV there are _____ (no / three) specific symptoms that must always be present for a diagnosis of schizophrenia to be made, nor is the presence of any _____ (one symptom / combination of symptoms) enough to diagnose schizophrenia. Rather, diagnoses are made based on the _____ (presence of several / lack of any) characteristic psychotic symptoms which occur in some combination with each other and have been active for a minimum of one _____ (month / year).

10-3	What is meant by positive symptoms of schizophrenia? What are they?

7.   In your own words, define the concept of positive symptoms as they relate to schizophrenia.

8.   a.   What are delusions?

    b.   What are two specific problems which sometimes make it difficult to decide if a belief is actually a delusion?

9. Match the following.

1. ____ somatic delusions
2. ____ delusions of persecution
3. ____ delusions of reference
4. ____ thought withdrawal
5. ____ thought insertion
6. ____ thought broadcasting
7. ____ delusions of grandeur

a. Camilla believes that there are insects under her skin consuming her internal organs.

b. Roberto suffers from delusions of control; he believes that people can hear his thoughts.

c. Tony believes that he is Christ.

d. Tomika believes that aliens have been spying on her and trying to kill her.

e. Benjamin believes that any newspaper article which begins with the letter B is really about him, because his name also begins with a B.

f. This is a delusion of control where a person believes that other people have the ability to force thoughts into his or her mind.

g. This is a delusion of control where a person believes that other people have the ability to steal thoughts out of his or her mind.

10. a. What is an hallucination?

b. How are hallucinations different from illusions?

c. 1. What are the most common type of hallucinations reported by those with schizophrenia?

2.   Briefly describe other possible hallucinations.

11. Whereas _____ (mania and depression / delusions and hallucinations) are disturbances in the content of thoughts, _____ (formication / formal thought disorder) involve fundamental disturbances in the form of thought—in how thoughts are organized, controlled and processed. Because clinicians cannot directly observe how people think, they must infer thought processes from _____ (CAT scans / speech).

12. Match the following disorders of thought processing.

1.   ____ derailment, cognitive slippage or loose associations
2.   ____ word salad
3.   ____ neologisms
4.   ____ perseveration
5.   ____ clang associations

a.   Words which have meaning only to the speaker.

b.   A word or concept is repeated over and over.

c.   The speaker cannot maintain a specific train of thought.

d.   Extremely disorganized speech where words seem to be selected at random and don't fit together.

e.   Words are chosen not for what they mean, but because they sound alike.

13. In your own words, briefly describe the following disorders of behavior.

a.   catatonia

b.   disorganized behavior

c.   psychomotor disturbances

10-4   What is meant by negative symptoms of schizophrenia? What are they?

14. In your own words, define the concept of negative symptoms as they relate to schizophrenia.

15. In your own words, briefly describe the following negative symptoms which are among the criteria for diagnosing schizophrenia.

  a. flat affect

  b. alogia

  c. avolation

10-5   What are some of the other psychotic disorders and how do they differ from schizophrenia?

16. Fill in the missing information.

PSYCHOTIC DISORDER	TYPICAL FEATURES	HOW THIS DISORDER IS DIFFERENT FROM SCHIZOPHRENIA
Brief Psychotic Disorder		
Schizophreniform Disorder		
Schizoaffective Disorder		
Delusional Disorder		

Shared Psychotic Disorder		
Substance-Induced Psychotic Disorder		

10-6	What is the course of schizophrenia?

17. a.   What is the average age of people first admitted to a hospital because of schizophrenia?

b.   Is it possible for a person in their fifties or sixties to develop schizophrenia?

18. Although childhood-onset schizophrenia is rare, it can occur. In what two ways is childhood-onset schizophrenia different from autistic disorder?

a.

b.

19. In your own words, briefly describe the three possible phases of schizophrenia.

a.   prodromal phase

b.   active phase

c.   residual phase

10-7	Which persons are most likely to develop schizophrenia?

20. a. Using the DSM-IV criteria, about _____ (1 / 10) percent of the world's population suffers from schizophrenia. Schizophrenia is found in _____ (all / only a few) geographic areas and cultures, with patients from so-called developing or Third World countries showing _____ (higher / lower) rates of improvement than patients in other countries.

  b. Throughout the world, schizophrenia is found in _____ (all / only the poorest) social classes. In the United States, a disproportionately _____ (low / high) incidence of the disease comes from poorer persons living in inner cities.

  c. The risk of developing schizophrenia is _____ (equal for men and women / higher for women). However, the average age of first onset is at least five years earlier for _____ (males / females) than for _____ (males / females).

Test your understanding

1. _____ is a general term which refers to a serious mental disorder in which the individual lacks an accurate perception of reality.
   a. Neurosis
   b. Psychosis
   c. Anxiety
   d. Schizophrenia

2. Which of the following is not a pattern of disruption typically caused by schizophrenia?
   a. blunted or inappropriate emotion
   b. bizarre and outlandish behavior
   c. disorganized and confused thinking
   d. attention level so focused that it is difficult to focus on something new

3. Who coined the term schizophrenia and categorized the symptoms as either primary or secondary?
   a. Benedict Morel
   b. Emil Kraepelin
   c. Eugen Bleuler
   d. Kurt Schneider

4. Positive symptoms of schizophrenia
   a. are distortions in normal psychological functioning which produce excesses in behavior.
   b. involve a lessening, absence or loss of normal functioning.
   c. are symptoms which actually aid the person in functioning, such as heightened levels of creativity.
   d. are symptoms which show up as a positive response on diagnostic questionnaires for schizophrenia.

5. Delusional beliefs in which the person misinterprets various stimuli as having special reference only to them are called
   a. delusions of control.
   b. delusions of reference.
   c. delusions of persecution.
   d. somatic delusions.

6. Thought withdrawal, thought insertion and thought broadcasting are all
   a. delusions of control.
   b. delusions of reference.
   c. delusions of persecution.
   d. somatic delusions.

7. Which are the most common type of hallucinations reported by those with schizophrenia?
   a. visual hallucinations
   b. tactile hallucinations
   c. auditory hallucinations
   d. olfactory hallucinations

8. A schizophrenic patient makes the following statement, "The summerbums of my repidicular pants are quite rawful." This is an example of
   a. catatonia.
   b. neologisms.
   c. clang associations.
   d. flat affect.

9. Disordered behavior, which can range from immobility to extreme activity and agitated excitement, is termed
   a. catatonia.
   b. neologisms.
   c. clang associations.
   d. flat affect.

10. What are negative symptoms of schizophrenia?
   a. They are distortions in normal psychological functioning which produce excesses in behavior.
   b. They involve a lessening, absence or loss of normal functioning.
   c. They are symptoms which cause problems in a person's life.
   d. They are symptoms which show up as a negative response on diagnostic questionnaires for schizophrenia.

11. A common symptom of schizophrenia which includes an emotionless state where the person stares straight ahead with a glazed unresponsive look is called
   a. alogia.
   b. schizophrenic stupor.
   c. inappropriate affect.
   d. flat affect.

12. A psychotic disorder in which symptoms begin suddenly, usually following an extreme stressor and last from one day to less than a month is called
   a. brief psychotic disorder.
   b. schizophreniform disorder.
   c. schizoaffective disorder.
   d. delusional disorder.

13. A psychotic disorder in which hallucinations and delusions are present along with episodes of mania and/or depression is called
   a. brief psychotic disorder.
   b. schizophreniform disorder.
   c. schizoaffective disorder.
   d. delusional disorder.

14. For over a year, Michael has been slowly sinking into schizophrenia. He is becoming more and more socially and emotionally withdrawn; his self-care activities are slipping and he is showing other negative symptoms. Michael has never shown these symptoms before. Which phase of schizophrenia best describes Michael's condition?
   a. the prodromal phase
   b. the active phase
   c. the passive phase
   d. the residual phase

15. Schizophrenia affects approximately what percentage of the world's population?
   a. 1 percent
   b. 5 percent
   c. 10 percent
   d. 15 percent

Answers to test your understanding

1. b. (10-1)
2. d. (10-1)
3. c. (10-1)
4. a. (10-2)
5. b. (10-3)
6. a. (10-3)
7. c. (10-3)
8. b. (10-3)
9. a. (10-3)
10. b. (10-4)
11. d. (10-4)
12. a. (10-5)
13. c. (10-5)
14. a. (10-6)
15. a. (10-7)

10-8   How is schizophrenia divided into subtypes by the DSM-IV and other classification systems?

---

21. Why do many clinicians refer to this disorder as the schizophrenias rather than schizophrenia?

22. Match the following.

1. ____ paranoid type schizophrenia
2. ____ disorganized type schizophrenia
3. ____ catatonic type schizophrenia
4. ____ undifferentiated type schizophrenia
5. ____ residual type schizophrenia

a. This is the most commonly used diagnostic category, utilized in cases where the basic criteria for schizophrenia are met; but they do not satisfy the specific criteria for paranoid, disorganized or catatonic subtypes.

b. The defining symptoms are prominent, persistent and elaborate delusions, usually involving themes of persecution. Auditory hallucinations, which are related to the delusional beliefs, are often present.

c. This category is used to describe situations where a patient has had at least one prior episode of schizophrenia, but does not currently display any major positive symptoms.

d.   This is a rare subtype, defined by extremely disordered, odd motor movements.

e.   This subtype is defined by grossly inappropriate and disorganized speech, behavior and affect (mood).

23. In your own words, briefly describe the following classifications of schizophrenia.

a.   process schizophrenia

b.   reactive schizophrenia

c.   Type I schizophrenia

d.   Type II schizophrenia

10-9	Is schizophrenia related to genetic factors?

24. Using the table below, indicate how family aggregation studies, twin studies and adoption studies either support or reject the following statements about the role of genetics in schizophrenia.

	SCHIZOPHRENIA "RUNS" IN FAMILIES, OFTEN BECAUSE VULNERABILITY TO THE DISORDER CAN BE GENETICALLY TRANSMITTED	GENES ALONE ARE NOT SUFFICIENT TO ACCOUNT FOR THE DEVELOPMENT OF SCHIZOPHRENIA
Family Aggregation Studies		
Twin Studies		

Adoption Studies		

25. a.   In the search for a genetic model of schizophrenia, many researchers today believe that the genetic contribution to the majority of cases of schizophrenia is polygenic. What does this mean?

    b.   Many authorities in the field believe that a diathesis-stress model probably best explains most cases of schizophrenia. Explain.

10-10   Is schizophrenia related to early physical trauma?

26. a.   Why do the findings of twin studies point to early physical trauma as a causal factor in some cases of schizophrenia?

    b.   What is the major suspected source of early physical trauma under investigation today? What are other possible sources of trauma?

10-11   How are the brains of those suffering from schizophrenia different in structure and function?

27. In your own words, briefly describe how each of the following brain structures may be involved in schizophrenic symptoms.

    a.   the frontal lobes

    b.   the temporal lobes and parts of the limbic system which lie underneath

c.   the thalamus

10-12   What is the role of biochemical processes in schizophrenia?

28. a.   Which neurotransmitter has received the most research support over the last forty years as a
potential causal factor in schizophrenia?

b.   Historically, what have scientists believed about this neurotransmitter?

c.   How do scientists today view the excess dopamine hypothesis as an explanation of the
relationship between neurotransmitters and schizophrenia?

| 10-13   What has been learned from the study of those people who are at risk for developing
schizophrenia? |
| --- |

29. a.   What are high-risk (HR) studies of schizophrenia?

b.   In your own words, summarize the major findings of high-risk studies.

10-14   How are social class and place of residence related to schizophrenia?

30. a.   In the United States, higher rates of schizophrenia are found among those living in
_____ (rural / urban) settings and members of the _____ (lower / middle / upper)
class.

b.   How do the following theories attempt to account for the statement above?

1.   social drift hypothesis

2.   social residue hypothesis

3.   breeder or social causation hypothesis

10-15   Is early family environment related to schizophrenia?

31. Decades ago, researchers described the schizophrenogenic mother and double-bind communication as causal factors in schizophrenia.

a.   In your own words, briefly describe these two theories.

b.   Are these theories taken seriously by researchers today?

c.   What problem has developed because of public acceptance of these theories?

10-16   Can the manner in which families express emotion be related to schizophrenia?

32. a.   In your own words, briefly describe the concept of expressed emotion (EE).

b.   Is expressed emotion related to the original onset of schizophrenia or relapses of it?

10-17   What biologically-based treatments are used to help control the symptoms of schizophrenia?

---

33.   The drugs most commonly used for schizophrenia are called antipsychotics or _____ (neuroleptics / schizoleptics). These drugs work by _____ (blocking / increasing) the action of the neurotransmitter _____ (serotonin / dopamine) in the brain.

34.   In your own words, briefly describe the following possible side effects of neuroleptic medications.

a.   Parkinsonism

b.   acute dystonia

c.   acute akathesia

d.   tardive dyskinesia

e.   neuroleptic malignant syndrome

35.   What is clozapine (Clozaril) and how does it affect the body?

10-18   What psychosocial treatments are used to help control the symptoms of
schizophrenia?

36. In your own words, briefly describe how each of the following are used in the treatment and
management of schizophrenia.

   a.   self-management and social skills training

   b.   family therapy

   c.   psychosocial rehabilitation

Test your understanding

1. Which subtype of schizophrenia is the most
commonly used category and describes
cases where the basic criteria for
schizophrenia are met, but do not satisfy the
specific criteria for paranoid, disorganized
or catatonic subtypes?
   a.   Type III schizophrenia
   b.   disorganized type schizophrenia
   c.   uncharacteristic type schizophrenia
   d.   undifferentiated type schizophrenia

2. Which subtype of schizophrenia involves
prominent, persistent and elaborate
delusions, usually involving themes of
persecution often accompanied by auditory
hallucinations?
   a.   paranoid type schizophrenia
   b.   disorganized type schizophrenia
   c.   catatonic type schizophrenia
   d.   undifferentiated type schizophrenia

3. Process schizophrenia
   a.   involves a rapid onset, usually
following a stressor, good premorbid
adjustment and a relatively good
prognosis.
   b.   involves slow deterioration, poor
premorbid adjustment and a relatively
poor prognosis.
   c.   is identical to Type I schizophrenia.
   d.   is identical to catatonic type
schizophrenia.

4. Type I schizophrenia
   a.   includes mostly positive symptoms.
   b.   includes mostly negative symptoms.
   c.   usually involves gradual onset.
   d.   is the new designation for dissociative
identify disorder (multiple personality
disorder).

5. Many researchers today believe that
    a. there is a single dominant gene which is responsible for the majority of cases of schizophrenia.
    b. there are two recessive genes which are responsible for the majority of cases of schizophrenia.
    c. different genes act together to influence the development, probability and severity of schizophrenia.
    d. genes are not related to the development, probability or severity of schizophrenia.

6. What is the major environmental trauma which is thought to be related to the development of some cases of schizophrenia?
    a. child abuse
    b. child neglect
    c. viral infection in early life
    d. accidents

7. Which of the following statements about the role of the frontal lobes in schizophrenia is not true?
    a. The frontal lobes are involved in planning, decision making and abstract thinking.
    b. The frontal lobes are often found to be decreased in volume and diminished in blood flow in schizophrenics.
    c. Irregularities with the frontal lobes may account for various negative symptoms.
    d. The only brain sites suspected of relating to schizophrenic symptoms are the frontal lobes.

8. Which neurotransmitter has received the most research support over the last forty years as a potential causal factor in schizophrenia?
    a. serotonin
    b. dopamine
    c. norepinephrine
    d. GABA

9. Today, the excess dopamine hypothesis
    a. is still considered to be the most accurate description of the role of neurotransmitters in schizophrenia.
    b. is thought to be too simplistic in its description of the role of neurotransmitters in schizophrenia.
    c. is no longer used, because of the undeserved guilt it caused for the families of schizophrenics.
    d. is no longer used, because researchers have proven that neurotransmitters are not involved in schizophrenia.

10. Which of the following statements about studies involving persons at high-risk (HR) for schizophrenia is not true?
    a. HR studies are based on a prospective design which follows participants from an early age to adulthood.
    b. HR studies focus on children thought to be predisposed to schizophrenia by virtue of having been born to a parent with schizophrenia.
    c. HR studies suggest that being born to a parent with schizophrenia is a reasonably good indicator of developing a serious psychological disorder, including schizophrenia.
    d. HR studies show that the vast majority of children born to schizophrenic parents go on to develop the disorder themselves.

11. In the United States, the highest rates of schizophrenia are found among
    a. the urban poor.
    b. urban dwellers of any social class.
    c. the rural poor.
    d. the suburban middle class.

12. The beliefs that the schizophrenogenic mother and double-bind communication patterns are significant causal factors for schizophrenia
    a. are firmly held by most researchers today.

b.   are supported by family studies.

c.   are supported by high-risk studies.

d.   have caused much undeserved blame and feelings of guilt for the family members of schizophrenics.

13.   Which of the following statements about the role of expressed emotion (EE) in schizophrenia is not true?

a.   EE describes problematic emotional exchanges between schizophrenic patients and their families.

b.   EE has been shown to be related to the original onset of schizophrenia.

c.   EE has been shown to be related to schizophrenic relapse.

d.   EE involves high levels of criticism, hostility and overinvolvement.

14.   Tardive dyskinesia is caused by

a.   long-term use of neuroleptic medications.

b.   overuse of ECT therapy.

c.   the same factors which cause schizophrenia.

d.   neuroleptic malignant syndrome.

15.   What is psychosocial rehabilitation?

a.   It is the training of necessary self-management and social skills to help schizophrenic patients deal with life in a mental institution. This training greatly enhances the effects of other forms of therapy.

b.   It is a program designed to educate the families of schizophrenics.

c.   It is a set of different interventions designed to prevent unnecessary hospitalizations, reduce impairments of daily functioning, strengthen daily living skills and increase social support for schizophrenic patients.

d.   It is a program designed to provide rest and rehabilitation for those working with schizophrenic patients.

Answers to test your understanding

1.   d.   (10-8)
2.   a.   (10-8)
3.   b.   (10-8)
4.   a.   (10-8)
5.   c.   (10-9)
6.   c.   (10-10)
7.   d.   (10-11)
8.   b.   (10-12)
9.   b.   (10-12)
10.   d.   (10-13)
11.   a.   (10-14)
12.   d.   (10-15)
13.   b.   (10-16)
14.   a.   (10-17)
15.   c.   (10-18)

When you have finished . . .

Explore the Web to find more information

An extremely comprehensive Web site is **The Schizophrenia Home Page**, which you can access at (**http://www.schizophrenia.com/**). Some of the links you will find there include:

> Current Schizophrenia News and Events
> On-Line Support Groups/Discussion Areas on Schizophrenia
> Discussion areas for problems and issues relating to Schizophrenia
> Information Area for Family and Friends of those with Schizophrenia
> Information Area for People who have Schizophrenia
> Information for Researchers and Industry Professionals
> Information for Students - Report/Writing Sources

The schizophrenia page from **Internet Mental Health** is loaded with information, articles and links. Go to (**http://www.mentalhealth.com/dis/p20-ps01.html**) to find it.

Another good starting point is **Doctor's Guide to Schizophrenia Information and Resources** at (**http://www.pslgroup.com/SCHIZOPHR.HTM#Disease**). The many links that you will find there can be divided into general information, medical news and alerts (you will find lots of in depth schizophrenia information here) and specific information about schizophrenia.

A publication from the **National Institutes of Mental Health**, "SCHIZOPHRENIA: Questions and Answers," can be accessed at (**http://www.nimh.nih.gov/publicat/schizo.htm**).

If you would like to see Positron Emission Tomography (PET) scans of blood flow in identical twins, one of whom has schizophrenia, go to (**http://www.nimh.nih.gov/research/sc6.htm**). These scans are provided by the **National Institutes of Mental Health.**

CHAPTER 11
Cognitive Disorders

Before you read . . .

Survey the chapter

Chapter 11 discusses the cognitive disorders. This a group of mental disorders that are directly caused by biological changes in the brain which impair higher level thinking processes such as memory, understanding, perception and recognition. Although cognitive disorders can occur at any age, they are especially common in older people.

The chapter begins with the case of Dorothy, a 78-year-old woman who is suffering from the insidious effects of Alzheimer's disease. The discussion then turns to the changes which normally occur with aging and how cognitive disorders are often associated with, but are not a natural part of the aging process. Amnestic disorders, delirium and dementia are then presented. The chapter concludes with an in depth discussion of the symptoms, possible causes and interventions for Alzheimer's disease.

As you read . . .

Ask questions

11-1   What is meant by the concept of cognitive disorders?

11-2   What physical and cognitive changes normally occur with aging?

11-3   What are some of the cognitive disorders related to aging?

11-4   What are the typical characteristics and patterns of amnestic disorders?

11-5   What are the typical characteristics and patterns of delirium?

11-6   What are the typical characteristics and patterns of dementia?

11-7   What medical conditions, other than Alzheimer's disease, can cause dementia?

11-8   What is Alzheimer's disease?

11-9   In what stages do the course of symptoms associated with Alzheimer's disease develop?

11-10   How does Alzheimer's disease affect brain structure?

11-11   Is Alzheimer's disease associated to genetic factors?

11-12   What factors, other than genetics, increase the risk for Alzheimer's disease?

11-13   Are there effective medical treatments for Alzheimer's disease?

11-14   How can caregivers of Alzheimer's patients best respond to patient needs?

After you read . . .

Review and explore the chapter

11-1   What is meant by the concept of cognitive disorders?

1.   The cognitive disorders are directly caused by _____ (psychosocial stressors / biological damage to the brain). They involve impairments in _____ (many different cognitive functions / memory) and can occur at any age, though they are especially common in _____ (infants / older people).

2.   a.   What is meant by focal damage to the brain?

   b.   What is meant by diffuse brain damage?

3.   The symptoms of cognitive disorders can take on many forms. List eight possibilities.

   a.

   b.

c.

d.

e.

f.

g.

h.

| 11-2 | What physical and cognitive changes normally occur with aging? |

4. What is ageism?

5. What does research tell us about commonly held beliefs about the aged, such as the belief that older persons have no interest in an active sex life, intellectual decline is inevitable and untreatable or that old age is a lonely, unhappy time?

6. a. What are the effects of aging on sensory and motor function?

b.   A number of metabolic changes occur with age. How can these changes influence the effects of medications on older persons?

c.   Respond to the statement, "Most older persons are unable to analyze and understand their daily experiences as well as when they were in their younger days."

d.   What are some possible reasons for memory loss in older persons other than the normal effects of aging?

11-3   What are some of the cognitive disorders related to aging?

---

7.   Match the following.

1.   ____ amnestic disorders
2.   ____ delirium
3.   ____ dementia
4.   ____ aphasia
5.   ____ agnosia
6.   ____ apraxia
7.   ____ disturbed executive functioning

a.   a disturbance in language

b.   memory loss without serious cognitive impairment

c.   often called senility by laypersons, involves loss of many cognitive abilities

d.   inability to recognize or interpret objects through one or more senses

e.   disturbance in consciousness that often develops rapidly and fluctuates dramatically

f.   inability to carry out motor activities, even though the necessary motor functions are intact

g.   loss of ability to plan or organize activities or to make good judgements

---

11-4	What are the typical characteristics and patterns of amnestic disorders?

8. Amnesia involves pure memory loss; if other cognitive failures are also prominent, _____ (delirium or dementia / no disorder) will usually be diagnosed. Amnestic disorders are caused by the direct effects of _____ (dissociation / a general medical condition) or the persisting effects of _____ (a substance / stress). In order to be diagnosed as an amnestic disorder, the memory loss must be serious enough to cause _____ (concern from the person / problems with functioning). The inability to learn new information is called _____ (anterograde amnesia / retrograde amnesia). The inability to recall information previously learned is called _____ (anterograde amnesia / retrograde amnesia).

9. What are three reasons why is it difficult to estimate the prevalence of amnestic disorders?

    a.

    b.

    c.

11-5	What are the typical characteristics and patterns of delirium?

10. Fill in the missing information about delirium in the table below.

DELIRIUM	
What is the typical course of onset in children?	
What is the typical course of onset in the elderly?	
What are the warning signs of an impending episode?	
What are the effects on consciousness?	

What are the effects on emotions?	
Can hallucinations and delusions occur in delirium?	
What are the effects on memory?	
Do cases of delirium run their course rapidly or slowly?	
Is complete recovery possible?	

11. Why is advanced age a risk factor for delirium?

12. What are some of the common causes of delirium?

13. In your own words, describe the major goal and associated factors which need to be addressed when treating delirium.

11-6   What are the typical characteristics and patterns of dementia?

14. a.   In your own words, briefly describe the major symptoms of dementia.

    b.   In what ways does dementia differ from delirium?

    c.   In what ways does dementia differ from depression?

11-7	What medical conditions, other than Alzheimer's disease, can cause dementia?

15. a.   What is vascular dementia?

b.   Is vascular dementia a common form of dementia?

c.   In what ways does vascular dementia differ from Alzheimer's disease?

16. Fill in the table below which lists other medical conditions which can cause dementia.

MEDICAL CONDITION	DESCRIPTION OF THE MEDICAL CONDITION
Pick's Disease	
Lewy Body Dementia	
Parkinson's Disease	
Huntington's Disease	
Creutzfeldt-Jakob Disease	
HIV Infection	
Syphilis	
Head Trauma	

Test your understanding

1. Cognitive disorders
   a. are caused by biological damage to the brain.
   b. are caused by psychosocial stressors.
   c. occur only in persons over age 65.
   d. affect only memory.

2. Which of the following is not one of the typical symptoms of cognitive disorders?
   a. inability to remember events that happened minutes before
   b. failure to recognize familiar people or objects
   c. profound confusion and disorientation
   d. loss of ability to understand speech while still comprehending written language

3. As people age
   a. body flexibility, muscle strength and speed remain relatively unaffected.
   b. the effects of drugs increase.
   c. the sensations of hearing, vision, smell and taste remain relatively unaffected.
   d. they lose the ability to understand and analyze the world around them.

4. Aphasia involves
   a. a disturbance in language.
   b. an inability to recognize or interpret objects through one or more senses.
   c. an inability to carry out motor activities, even though the necessary motor functions are intact.
   d. a loss of ability to plan or organize activities or to make good judgements.

5. Apraxia involves
   a. a disturbance in language.
   b. an inability to recognize or interpret objects through one or more senses.
   c. an inability to carry out motor activities, even though the necessary motor functions are intact.

d. a loss of ability to plan or organize activities or to make good judgements.

6. The inability to recall information previously learned is called
   a. anterograde amnesia.
   b. retrograde amnesia.
   c. delirium.
   d. dementia.

7. Which of the following statements about delirium is not true?
   a. The onset of delirium in children is often different than in the elderly.
   b. Delirium may include visual hallucinations and paranoid delusions.
   c. Memory for recent events is commonly impaired, while memory for events which happened long ago remains intact.
   d. The course of delirium is slow and chronic.

8. What is the major goal when treating delirium?
   a. provide reassurance to the patient
   b. provide reassurance to the family of the patient
   c. identify the underlying cause of the delirium
   d. increase the level of medication, until a therapeutic level is reached

9. Dementia
   a. includes the loss of cognitive functions to the point that it interferes with daily functioning.
   b. runs its course much more rapidly than delirium.
   c. is almost impossible to distinguish from depression when it occurs in older persons.
   d. is easily treated, once the underlying cause is determined.

10. Vascular dementia
    a. is the leading cause of dementia in persons over age 70.
    b. is caused by a series of strokes in the brain.
    c. is caused by a series of heart attacks.
    d. is almost impossible to distinguish from Alzheimer's disease when it occurs in older persons.

Answers to test your understanding

1. a. (11-1)
2. d. (11-1)
3. b. (11-2)
4. a. (11-3)
5. c. (11-3)
6. b. (11-4)
7. d. (11-5)
8. c. (11-5)
9. a. (11-6)
10. b. (11-7)

11-8   What is Alzheimer's disease?

---

17. Alzheimer's disease is by far the most frequent cause of dementia, accounting for over _____ (one-half / 90 percent) of cases seen in persons over age 65. Dementia of Alzheimer's type now affects more than _____ (one million / four million) Americans today. The incidence of dementia due to Alzheimer's disease _____ (doubles / quadruples) every 5 years of increased age between the ages of 65 and 85. When onset of dementia of the Alzheimer's type occurs before age 65, it is diagnosed as _____ (Type I Alzheimer's disease / with early onset). When onset occurs after age 65, which is much _____ (less / more) common, it is diagnosed as _____ (Type II Alzheimer's disease / with late onset).

11-9   In what stages do the course of symptoms associated with Alzheimer's disease develop?

---

18. In your own words, briefly outline both the common symptoms and problems in functioning associated with the three stages of Alzheimer's disease listed below.

    a. early stages

    b. middle stages

    c. later stages

19. What is the average life expectancy of an Alzheimer's patient after the onset of symptoms occurs?

11-10   How does Alzheimer's disease affect brain structure?

---

20. What areas of the brain show atrophy from the effects of Alzheimer's disease?

21. Name and describe the two most distinctive signs of brain damage due to Alzheimer's disease?

    a.

    b.

22. What is beta-amyloid-4 and how is it possibly related to Alzheimer's disease?

11-11   Is Alzheimer's disease associated to genetic factors?

---

23. Next to age, _____ (general health / family history), is one of the strongest risk factors for Alzheimer's disease. By the time individuals reach age 90, their risk of developing Alzheimer's disease is almost _____ (50 / 99) percent, if they had parents or siblings with the disease.

24. Fill in the missing information about the relationship of genetic factors to Alzheimer's disease, in the table below.

	TIED TO EARLY ONSET OR LATE ONSET?	EVIDENCE OF LINKAGE TO ALZHEIMER'S DISEASE
Chromosome 21		

Chromosome 1	no information	
Chromosome 14		
Chromosome 19		

11-12   What factors, other than genetics, increase the risk for Alzheimer's disease?

25. Explain why it is believed that the following may be related to an increased risk for Alzheimer's disease.

    a.   head trauma

    b.   coronary artery disease

    c.   environmental toxins

    d.   acetylcholine (ACh) deficiency

    e.   low levels of education

11-13   Are there effective medical treatments for Alzheimer's disease?

26. Why have there been problems in developing an effective medical treatment for Alzheimer's disease?

27. Match the following.

1. ____ Tacrine (COGNEX)
2. ____ estrogen
3. ____ Deprenyl (ELDEPRYL)
4. ____ vitamin E
5. ____ Nimodipine
6. ____ Propentofylline
7. ____ anti-inflammatory agents

   a. destroys MAO-B

   b. As of 1995, this was the only drug with FDA approval to treat Alzheimer's disease. It
       slows the breakdown of ACh.

   c. promotes synapse formation and increases ACh synthesis

   d. blocks inflammatory responses in hopes of reducing neural damage

   e. a calcium channel blocker, it slows the progression of Alzheimer's disease because calcium
       aids in the degeneration of neurons

   f. enhances blood flow and energy metabolism in the brain

   g. inactivates oxygen free radicals, a source of damage to neurons

---

| 11-14 | How can caregivers of Alzheimer's patients best respond to patient needs? |

28. Because Alzheimer's disease is a chronic condition for which a cure is not available, long-term care is
     focused on the management of the patient's symptoms and behavior. In your own words, briefly
     discuss three factors which are important for the caregivers of Alzheimer's disease patients to
     remember.

   a.

   b.

   c.

Test your understanding

1. By far, the most frequent cause of dementia is
   a. Pick's disease.
   b. Huntington's disease.
   c. Creutzfeldt-Jakob disease.
   d. Alzheimer's disease.

2. Early onset Alzheimer's disease
   a. is more common than late onset type.
   b. describes an onset of symptoms before age 45.
   c. describes an onset of symptoms before age 65.
   d. is not nearly as disabling as the late onset type.

3. Which of the following statements about Alzheimer's disease is not true?
   a. In the early stages of Alzheimer's disease, the primary symptoms are increased forgetfulness and loss of the ability to cope with change.
   b. In the middle stages of Alzheimer's disease, the primary symptoms are increased problems with language, understanding and perception.
   c. In the later stages of Alzheimer's disease, the primary symptoms are loss of language and an inability to function even in familiar places.
   d. In the last stage of Alzheimer's disease, the person tends to gain back some of the lost functions and abilities for short periods, especially at night.

4. The two most distinctive signs of brain damage due to Alzheimer's disease are
   a. neurofibrillary tangles and neuritic plaques.
   b. vascular and hormonal damage.
   c. fewer neurons and plaques.
   d. increased number of neurons and plaques.

5. Next to age, _____ is one of the strongest risk factors for Alzheimer's disease.
   a. blood type
   b. education level
   c. family history
   d. stress

6. Which chromosome has been linked to late onset Alzheimer's disease?
   a. 21
   b. 1
   c. 14
   d. 19

7. Which of the following is not related to increased risk for Alzheimer's disease?
   a. head trauma
   b. growing up in a rural environment
   c. exposure to environmental toxins
   d. low levels of education

8. Why have there been problems in developing an effective medical treatment for Alzheimer's disease?
   a. Because clinicians do not know enough about the causes of the disease or the biological mechanisms leading to cell death to develop interventions which are effective.
   b. Because of the ageism present in most Western cultures, most researchers would rather focus on diseases of the young.
   c. Because the aging process causes so many other problems, it makes it difficult to separate and focus on the specific symptoms of Alzheimer's disease.
   d. Because most Alzheimer's disease patients and their families refuse treatment.

9. Tacrine is
    a. a famous treatment clinic, which treats Alzheimer's disease patients.
    b. a drug used to treat the symptoms of Alzheimer's disease.
    c. one of the four known causes of Alzheimer's disease.
    d. an abnormal protein found in the blood of early onset Alzheimer's disease patients.

10. It is important for the caregivers of Alzheimer's disease patients to do all of the following except
    a. respond to the patient's immediate emotional, psychological and physical needs.
    b. respond to the patient's need for emotional and physical closeness.
    c. talk to the patient in long and complex sentences, because verbal stimulation is important.
    d. remember that they need special help themselves.

Answers to test your understanding

1. d.   (11-8)
2. c.   (11-8)
3. d.   (11-9)
4. a.   (11-10)
5. c.   (11-11)
6. d.   (11-11)
7. b.   (11-12)
8. a.   (11-13)
9. b.   (11-13)
10. c.   (11-14)

When you have finished . . .

Explore the Web to find more information

Columbia Presbyterian Hospital provides the document, "Screening for Dementia." You can access it at (http://cait.cpmc.columbia.edu/texts/gcps/gcps047.html).

One of the best resources for information on Alzheimer's disease is the **Alzheimer's Association** Web site which is located at (http://www.alz.org/). Some of the many links they offer include:

What's New
General Information
Chapter Information
Caregiver Resources
Medical Information
Public Policy
Media Releases
Position statements
Green-Field Library
Related Resources

The **Michigan Alzheimer's Disease Research Center** offers a wide array of services and information. The URL is (**http://www.med.umich.edu/madrc/MADRC.html**).

The **Alzheimer Web** is devoted to research on Alzheimer's disease. You can find it by going to (**http://werple.mira.net.au/~dhs/ad.html**).

The following are articles on Alzheimer's disease.

- "Alzheimer's Disease." This comprehensive article is from the **National Institutes of Health's** Decade of the Brain Series. (**http://www.nimh.nih.gov/publicat/alzheim.htm**).

- "Cognitive Tests 90% Accurate in Predicting Alzheimer's," The Medical Post, April 9, 1996. This article, made available through **Internet Mental Health**, directly relates to the controversy box in this chapter. (**http://www.mentalhealth.com/mag1/p5m-alz3.html**)

Another informative publication by the **National Institutes of Health** is, "If You're Over 65 And Feeling Depressed. . . ." The URL is (**http://www.nimh.nih.gov/publicat/over65.htm**).

LewyNet is a WWW information source in England for those interested in Lewy body dementia. Accsess them at (**http://www.ccc.nottingham.ac.uk/~mpzjlowe/lewy/lewyhome.html**).

CHAPTER 12
Personality Disorders

Before you read . . .

Survey the chapter

Chapter 12 will introduce you to a category of disorders which is very different from any that you have yet encountered in your text. The disorders that you have studied so far are categorized in the DSM-IV as Axis I disorders, where symptoms intermittently disrupt otherwise healthy functioning. This chapter discusses Axis II disorders, problems in functioning which are an integral part of the person's personality structure. These are disorders where long-standing, extreme and rigid personality traits are maladaptive.

You will examine ten different personality disorders in this chapter. Some of the personality disorders revolve around behavioral characteristics which can be described as odd and eccentric, some as dramatic emotional and erratic, and some as fearful and anxious. The various disorders will be described and their causes and attempts at treatment will be discussed.

As you read . . .

Ask questions

12-1   What are the characteristics of personality disorders?

12-2   What are some of the problems encountered in diagnosing personality disorders?

12-3   What are the dimensions of personality disorders?

12-4   What are the characteristics of paranoid personality disorder?

12-5   What are the characteristics of schizoid personality disorder?

12-6   What are the characteristics of schizotypal personality disorder?

12-7   What are the characteristics of histrionic personality disorder?

12-8   What are the characteristics of narcissistic personality disorder?

12-9   What are the characteristics of borderline personality disorder?

12-10   What are the characteristics of antisocial personality disorder?

12-11   What are the characteristics of avoidant personality disorder?

12-12   What are the characteristics of dependent personality disorder?

12-13   What are the characteristics of obsessive-compulsive personality disorder?

12-14   Do genes dictate personality differences and influence personality disorders?

12-15   Can psychodynamic or interpersonal theory explain personality differences and personality disorders?

12-16   Can evolutionary theory explain personality differences and personality disorders?

12-17   What factors are related to the development of borderline personality disorder?

12-18   What factors are related to the development of antisocial personality disorder?

12-19   Can personality disorders be treated?

12-20   What is the most effective intervention used in the treatment of borderline personality disorder?

12-21   Are there effective interventions for the treatment of antisocial personality disorder?

After you read . . .

Review and explore the chapter

12-1   What are the characteristics of personality disorders?

1. The unique pattern of behavior which distinguishes each person from every other is called _____ (personality / ego-syntonic behavior). A particular attribute of a person's overall stable characteristic is called a _____ (personality trait / ego-syntonic factor). In the DSM-IV, personality disorders are placed on Axis _____ (I / II / III). In order to diagnose a personality disorder, an individual's personality traits must be _____ (overly flexible / maladaptive).

2. The long-term ingrained patterns of behavior seen in personality disorders are related to four other important features. What are they?

    a.

b.

c.

d.

3. a.   At what point in a person's life do personality disorders first become apparent?

b.   Although it is difficult to estimate, about what percentage of the population of the United States have met the criteria for at least one type of personality disorder at some time in their lives?

c.   Are most personality disorders diagnosed in men or women?

12-2   What are some of the problems encountered in diagnosing personality disorders?

4. a.   Is it possible for Axis II personality disorders to be comorbid with Axis I disorders?

b.   In your own words, briefly discuss three possible ways in which personality disorders may be related to Axis I disorders.

1.

2.

3.

5.   In your own words, briefly discuss three problems, other than comorbidity, which may make the diagnosis of personality disorders difficult.

a.

b.

c.

| 12-3 | What are the dimensions of personality disorders? |

6.   The factors from the Big Five model are listed below. Match each of them to the example which would probably indicate a low score for that factor.

1.   ____ neuroticism
2.   ____ extroversion
3.   ____ openness
4.   ____ agreeableness
5.   ____ conscientiousness

a.   Harry likes his job as a lighthouse keeper because its quiet and most of all, he doesn't have to deal with other people.

b.   You can never rely on Ann for anything. She doesn't seem to care that she is always late, careless and undependable.

    c.   Ramon is constantly anxious, Tomika is always angry about something and Chris is always unhappy. The one thing they do share is that their negative emotions disrupt their thinking and behavior.

    d.   Shane's consistently rude behavior is tied to his belief that everyone is out to take advantage of him or demean him in some way.

    e.   Pat is usually quite flat emotionally and has a long-established and inflexible way of doing things.

7.   In your own words, briefly describe Leary's Interpersonal Circumplex model of personality.

12-4	What are the characteristics of paranoid personality disorder?

8.   In your own words, briefly describe the major characteristics of paranoid personality disorder.

9.   What is the estimated prevalence of paranoid personality disorder in the United States?

12-5	What are the characteristics of schizoid personality disorder?

10.   In your own words, briefly describe the major characteristics of schizoid personality disorder.

11.   What is the estimated prevalence of schizoid personality disorder in the United States?

12-6	What are the characteristics of schizotypal personality disorder?

12.   In your own words, briefly describe the major characteristics of schizotypal personality disorder.

13. What is the estimated prevalence of schizotypal personality disorder in the United States?

| 12-7 | What are the characteristics of histrionic personality disorder? |

14. In your own words, briefly describe the major characteristics of histrionic personality disorder.

15. What is the estimated prevalence of histrionic personality disorder in the United States?

| 12-8 | What are the characteristics of narcissistic personality disorder? |

16. In your own words, briefly describe the major characteristics of narcissistic personality disorder.

17. What is the estimated prevalence of narcissistic personality disorder in the United States?

| 12-9 | What are the characteristics of borderline personality disorder? |

18. In your own words, briefly describe the major characteristics of borderline personality disorder.

19. a.   What is the estimated prevalence of borderline personality disorder in the United States?

b.   Is borderline personality disorder diagnosed more often in men or women?

12-10   What are the characteristics of antisocial personality disorder?

20. What are some of the earlier labels for what is now called antisocial personality disorder?

21. In your own words, briefly describe the major characteristics of antisocial personality disorder.

22. How does conduct disorder relate to antisocial personality disorder?

23. a.   What is the estimated prevalence of antisocial personality disorder in the United States?

    b.   Is antisocial personality disorder diagnosed more often in men or women?

Test your understanding

1. The unique pattern of behavior which distinguishes each person from every other is called
   a. personality.
   b. a personality disorder.
   c. ego-syntonic behavior.
   d. Axis II behavior.

2. In the DSM-IV, personality disorders are listed on Axis
   a. I.
   b. II.
   c. III.
   d. IV.

3. Which of the following statements about personality disorders is not true?
   a. Personality disorders tend to be ego-syntonic.
   b. Personality disorders are very difficult to treat.
   c. Personality disorders are usually very distressing to the person displaying them.
   d. It is estimated that between 10 and 13 percent of the United Stated population have met the criteria for at least one personality disorder at some point in their lives.

4. It is common for personality disorders to become apparent during
    a. infancy.
    b. middle childhood (ages 7-10).
    c. adolescence or early adulthood.
    d. middle adulthood (around age 40).

5. Are personality disorders often comorbid with Axis I disorders?
    a. No, because DSM-IV criteria demands that the presence of an Axis I disorder precludes a diagnosis of personality disorder.
    b. No, because DSM-IV criteria demands that the presence of a personality disorder precludes a diagnosis of Axis I disorders.
    c. Yes, because a person with a personality disorder always has comorbid Axis I problems.
    d. Yes, because the symptoms of personality disorders and Axis I disorders often overlap and/or influence each other.

6. On which factor on the Big Five model does a high score signify compassionate interest, concern and caring for others, while a low score indicates a tendency toward competitiveness, manipulation, hostility and rudeness?
    a. neuroticism
    b. agreeableness
    c. extroversion
    d. conscientiousness

7. On which factor on the Big Five model does a high score signify emotional stability and calmness while under stress, while a low score indicates a tendency toward negative emotions such as anxiety, anger and depression?
    a. neuroticism
    b. agreeableness
    c. extroversion
    d. conscientiousness

8. Which personality disorder involves long standing traits of suspiciousness and mistrust of others?
    a. paranoid personality disorder
    b. schizoid personality disorder
    c. schizotypal personality disorder
    d. antisocial personality disorder

9. Which personality disorder involves an indifference to social relationships and needs, as well as emotional flatness?
    a. paranoid personality disorder
    b. schizoid personality disorder
    c. schizotypal personality disorder
    d. antisocial personality disorder

10. Which personality disorder involves odd patterns of behavior, language, thinking and beliefs?
    a. paranoid personality disorder
    b. schizoid personality disorder
    c. schizotypal personality disorder
    d. antisocial personality disorder

11. Which personality disorder involves attention-getting behaviors which may include seductiveness, exaggerated displays of emotion and demands for reassurance and praise?
    a. histrionic personality disorder
    b. narcissistic personality disorder
    c. borderline personality disorder
    d. antisocial personality disorder

12. Which personality disorder involves an overinflated sense of self-importance and a preoccupation with special privilege and entitlement?
    a. histrionic personality disorder
    b. narcissistic personality disorder
    c. borderline personality disorder
    d. antisocial personality disorder

13. Which personality disorder is involved with impulsivity and instability in mood, behavior, self-image and interpersonal relationships? It is diagnosed more often in

women than in men.
a. histrionic personality disorder
b. narcissistic personality disorder
c. borderline personality disorder
d. antisocial personality disorder

14. Which personality disorder involves impulsivity, unreliability, insincerity when dealing with others, a disregard for the truth, lack of remorse, inability to learn from past mistakes and an inability to feel genuine emotion? It is diagnosed more often in men than in women.
a. histrionic personality disorder
b. narcissistic personality disorder
c. borderline personality disorder
d. antisocial personality disorder

15. A disorder, which often precedes and is similar to antisocial personality disorder, but occurs before age fifteen is
a. psychopathy.
b. sociopathy.
c. conduct disorder.
d. moral insanity.

Answers to test your understanding

1. a. (12-1)
2. b. (12-1)
3. c. (12-1)
4. c. (12-1)
5. d. (12-2)
6. b. (12-3)
7. a. (12-3)
8. a. (12-4)
9. b. (12-5)
10. c. (12-6)
11. a. (12-7)
12. b. (12-8)
13. c. (12-9)
14. d. (12-10)
15. c. (12-11)

| 12-11 | What are the characteristics of avoidant personality disorder? |

24. In your own words, briefly describe the major characteristics of avoidant personality disorder.

25. What is the estimated prevalence of avoidant personality disorder in the United States?

| 12-12 | What are the characteristics of dependent personality disorder? |

26. In your own words, briefly describe the major characteristics of dependent personality disorder.

27. What is the estimated prevalence of dependent personality disorder in the United States?

12-13   What are the characteristics of obsessive-compulsive personality disorder?

28. In your own words, briefly describe the major characteristics of obsessive-compulsive personality disorder.

29. What is the estimated prevalence of obsessive-compulsive personality disorder in the United States?

30. How does obsessive-compulsive personality disorder differ from the Axis I disorder, obsessive-compulsive disorder?

12-14   Do genes dictate personality differences and influence personality disorders?

31. Of nonshared environment, shared environment and genetic influence,

    a.   the most influential factor in determining personality characteristics is _____.

    b.   the next most influential factor in determining personality characteristics is _____.

    c.   the least influential factor in determining personality characteristics is _____.

32. For each of the personality disorders below, indicate if present research strongly supports, somewhat supports or has obtained mixed results, or does not support the role of genetics as a causal factor.

    a.   paranoid personality disorder   _____

    b.   schizoid personality disorder   _____

    c.   schizotypal personality disorder   _____

    d.   antisocial personality disorder   _____

e.   borderline personality disorder   _____

f.   narcissistic personality disorder   _____

g.   histrionic personality disorder   _____

h.   avoidant personality disorder   _____

i.   dependent personality disorder   _____

j.   obsessive-compulsive personality disorder _____

12-15   Can psychodynamic or interpersonal theory explain personality differences and personality disorders?

---

33. a.   In your own words, briefly describe how traditional psychodynamic theory attempted to explain personality disorders.

b.   Does this view receive much support from clinicians today?

34. In your own words, briefly describe how more recent psychodynamic formulations, such as those based on object relations theory, attempt to explain personality disorders.

35. In your own words, briefly describe how interpersonal learning theories attempt to explain personality disorders.

12-16   Can evolutionary theory explain personality differences and personality disorders?

---

36. a.   What are the three fundamental polarities which are the basis of Millon's evolutionary theory of personality?

1.

2.

3.

b.   How do these polarities relate to personality disorders?

12-17   What factors are related to the development of borderline personality disorder?

---

37. In your own words, briefly discuss the possible role of each of the following as a causal factor in borderline personality disorder.

a.   biological factors

b.   psychoanalytic factors

c.   early childhood trauma

12-18   What factors are related to the development of antisocial personality disorder?

---

38. Each of the following statements about biologically-based factors which may relate to the development of antisocial personality disorder is false. Correct each statement.

a.   Antisocial personality disorder seems to be related to an overdeveloped cerebral cortex. This may help explain problems with impulsive behavior.

b.   Persons with antisocial personality disorder tend to have unusually high levels of anxiety and physiological arousal.

c. Persons with antisocial personality disorder are probably predisposed biologically to quickly learn fear responses.

39. List five specific family variables which have been associated with antisocial behavior.

a.

b.

c.

d.

e.

12-19   Can personality disorders be treated?

---

40. In general, personality disorders are among the _____ (least problematic/ most difficult) mental disorders to treat, especially because of their status as a _____ (consistently shifting / long-standing) lifestyle. Traditional forms of psychotherapy _____ (are / are not) well suited for treating these problems. New, more specific approaches such as *self psychology*, which is used in the treatment of _____ (paranoid / narcissistic) personality disorder, are being developed. Substantial improvement has been obtained for avoidant personality disorder with _____ (drug / cognitive-behavioral) therapy.

12-20   What is the most effective intervention used in the treatment of borderline personality disorder?

---

41. In your own words, briefly describe the focus and format of dialectical behavior therapy (DBT) as it

is used to treat borderline personality disorder.

12-21   Are there effective interventions for the treatment of antisocial personality disorder?

---

42. a.   Are there effective interventions for the treatment of antisocial personality disorder?

b.   Why?

Test your understanding

1.   Which personality disorder is involved with a solitary lifestyle imposed by consistent feelings of inadequacy and ineptitude, especially in social situations?
     a.   antisocial personality disorder
     b.   avoidant personality disorder
     c.   dependent personality disorder
     d.   obsessive-compulsive personality disorder

2.   Which personality disorder involves such a lack of self-confidence that the person clings to others hoping for reassurance and information on how to conduct his or her life?
     a.   antisocial personality disorder
     b.   avoidant personality disorder
     c.   dependent personality disorder
     d.   obsessive-compulsive personality disorder

3.   Which personality disorder involves a rigid preoccupation with rules, details and minute organization and planning of every aspect of one's life?
     a.   antisocial personality disorder
     b.   avoidant personality disorder

       c.   dependent personality disorder
       d.   obsessive-compulsive personality disorder

4.   Are obsessive-compulsive personality disorder and obsessive-compulsive disorder (OCD) the same thing?
       a.   Yes, they are identical in all respects.
       b.   Yes, the symptoms are identical, but the causes are different.
       c.   No, obsessive-compulsive personality disorder describes a chronic lifestyle, as opposed to the specific obsessions and compulsions of OCD.
       d.   No, obsessive-compulsive personality disorder is listed as an Axis I disorder in the DSM-IV, while OCD is listed on Axis II.

5.   Which of the following probably had the most influence on the development of your personality characteristics?
       a.   your genetic makeup
       b.   your socioeconomic status
       c.   your birth order
       d.   your prenatal environment

6. Which of the following personality disorders is probably most influenced by genetic factors?
   a. avoidant personality disorder
   b. dependent personality disorder
   c. histrionic personality disorder
   d. antisocial personality disorder

7. Which of the following explanations of the causes of personality disorders has the least support from researchers and clinicians?
   a. genetic predisposition
   b. traditional psychodynamic theory
   c. more recent psychodynamic formulations
   d. object relations theory

8. Object relations theory emphasizes
   a. Freud's psychosexual stages.
   b. how people relate to the objects in their lives.
   c. attachments between infants and caretakers and later expectations for relationships.
   d. frontal lobe damage.

9. Which of the following is not one of Millon's three fundamental evolutionary polarities?
   a. the minimization of pain and the maximization of pleasure
   b. adapting to environmental demands through passive accommodation or active modification
   c. the desire to strengthen social bonds over avoidance and isolation
   d. advancing the self and caring for others

10. All of the following have been viewed as a plausible contributor to borderline personality disorder except
    a. organic brain problems.
    b. problems in the construction of self-identity during the first years of life.
    c. early childhood sexual or physical abuse.
    d. alcohol dependency.

11. The development of antisocial personality disorder may be related to
    a. an overdeveloped cerebral cortex.
    b. low levels of anxiety and physiological arousal.
    c. an overabundance of learned fear responses.
    d. alcohol dependency.

12. All of the following family variables have been linked to antisocial personality disorder except
    a. history of parental criminality.
    b. parental uninvolvement, erratic discipline, physical abuse or poor supervision of children.
    c. living in an urban area.
    d. exposure to deviant peers.

13. Personality disorders are among the most difficult to treat because
    a. they are extremely rare, so most clinicians have no experience dealing with them.
    b. most therapeutic techniques require a long-term effort and many persons with personality disorders can't financially afford to stay in treatment that long.
    c. the symptoms of personality disorders are long-standing lifestyles.
    d. none of the symptoms of personality disorders are directly observable.

14. The most effective psychotherapy for borderline personality disorder is
    a. dialectical behavior therapy.
    b. hypnosis, coupled with assertiveness skills training.
    c. traditional psychoanalysis.
    d. stress reduction skills training.

15. Is there an effective treatment for antisocial personality disorder?
    a. yes, traditional psychoanalysis
    b. yes, stress reduction skills training
    c. yes, dialectical behavior therapy
    d. no

Answers to test your understanding

1. b. (12-11)
2. c. (12-12)
3. d. (12-13)
4. c. (12-13)
5. a. (12-14)
6. d. (12-14)
7. b. (12-15)
8. c. (12-15)
9. c. (12-16)
10. d. (12-17)
11. b. (12-18)
12. c. (12-18)
13. c. (12-19)
14. a. (12-20)
15. d. (12-21)

When you have finished . . .

Explore the Web to find more information

The article, "The Roots of Personality: Heredity and Environment," by John E. Gedo, M.D., The Harvard Mental Health Letter, July, 1990 is provided by **Internet Mental Health** and can be accessed at (**http://www.mentalhealth.com/mag1/p5h-per2.html**).

Internet Mental Health articles on personality disorders include:

- (**http://www.mentalhealth.com/mag1/p5h-per1.html**) "Personality and Personality Disorders," The Harvard Medical School Mental Health Letter, September (Part I), October, 1987 (Part II).

- (**http://www.mentalhealth.com/mag1/p5h-per3.html**) "Personality Disorders: The Anxious Cluster," The Harvard Mental Health Letter, February (Part I), March, 1996 (Part II).

- (**http://www.mentalhealth.com/mag1/p5h-pe01.html**) "Psychopaths: New Trends in Research," by Robert D. Hare, The Harvard Mental Health Letter, September, 1995.

- (**http://www.mentalhealth.com/mag1/p5h-bor1.html**) "Borderline Sexuality," The Harvard Medical School Mental Health Letter, September, 1987 .

A number of resources dealing with borderline personality disorders are provided by **BPD Central**. They can be accessed at (**http://members.aol.com/BPDCentral/index.html**).

An article about one form of treatment for borderline personality, provided by **Psychiatry On-line**, is "An Overview of Dialectical Behaviour Therapy in the Treatment of Borderline Personality Disorder," by Barry Kiehn and Michaela Swales.   (**http://www.cityscape.co.uk/users/ad88/dbt1.htm**)

CHAPTER 13
Substance-Related Disorders

Before you read . . .

Survey the chapter

    Chapter 13 discusses issues dealing with the use and abuse of chemical substances. The chapter opens with the case of Jerry, a college student who is both confused and concerned about his increasing use of alcohol and other drugs. Basic terms and concepts as well as the DSM-IV criteria for describing and diagnosing substance use disorders are presented.

    A significant portion of this chapter is devoted to a discussion of alcohol use and alcohol use disorders. This includes an overview of the prevalence of alcohol use disorders, the effects of alcohol on the body and behavior and specific disorders associated with alcohol abuse. The causes, treatments and prevention of alcohol use disorders are also presented. The remainder of this chapter discusses the use and abuse of other psychoactive drugs, including depressants, stimulants, opiates, cannabis, hallucinogens and nicotine.

As you read . . .

Ask questions

13- 1   What are psychoactive drugs and what effects do they have on society? *Affect user's thinking, emotions & behavior; widely available & used by many - alcohol,*

13- 2   What terms and concepts are used to describe substance use and substance abuse?

13- 3   How does the DSM-IV describe substance related disorders?

13- 4   What do we know about alcohol abuse patterns in the United States?

13- 5   How does alcohol affect the body and behavior?

13- 6   What do we know about the prevalence of alcohol use disorders?

13- 7   How do we describe patterns of alcohol abuse?

13- 8   What other problems are associated with alcohol abuse and dependence?

13- nicotine & caffeine ② legally available through prescription - barbiturates, benzodiazepines, some opioids, and illegal cocaine, marijuana, LSD.

229

13- 9   What are the possible causes of alcohol use disorders?

13-10   How are alcohol use disorders treated?

13-11   What are depressants? How do they affect the body and behavior? How can depressant abuse and dependence be treated?

13-12   What are stimulants? How do they affect the body and behavior? How can stimulant abuse and dependence be treated?

13-13   What are opiates? How do they affect the body and behavior? How can opiate abuse and dependence be treated?

13-14   What are the effects of cannabis and hallucinogens? How are they abused and how are problems associated with these substances treated?

After you read . . .

Review and explore the chapter

13-1 What are psychoactive drugs and what effects do they have on society?

1.   What is a psychoactive drug? Define the term in your own words. ~~Because~~ They affect user's thinking, emotions & behavior.

2.   What is meant by the statement, "Many societies, including that of the United States, hold conflicting attitudes toward most substances?" Can you think of examples?

Billions of $ are spent manufacturing, advertising & selling drugs like alcohol & ~~caffeine~~ medicine, while at the same time, billions of $ are spent treating diseases, punishing crime, making up for absenteeism, etc, which are caused by drug abuse.

3.   What are three different ways that illegal drug use has had a negative impact in the United States?

a. About 375, 000 infants are born annually w/ mental or physical problems caused by in utero exposure to alcohol or drugs.
~~-9 negative prenatal effects on children~~

b. At least 3% of all deaths are directly linked to alcohol
~~-9 deaths directly linked to drugs~~

c. Criminal activities of each daily heroin user drains about $55,000/year from the economy + increase in criminal activities

---

13-2   What terms and concepts are used to describe substance use and substance abuse?

4. a. Describe four possible indications that drug use is actually drug abuse.

1. Level of use is hazardous to a persons health

2. Leads to significant impairment in work or family life

3. Produces personal distress

4. Leads to legal problems

b. Which is more important in determining when drug use has progressed to drug abuse, the amount consumed or the presence of adverse consequences from drug use?

Adverse consequence.

5. What three factors indicate psychological dependence? A/K/A dependence

a. desire/craving for the drug

b. increased time procuring & using drugs, reduced time for work, school, family, etc.

c. Continue to Consume drug, even when the user knows that it is causing problems

6. a. What is physiological dependence? A/HA addiction

This occurs when physical changes are brought on by excessive + frequent use of a substance

b. What two physical changes occur with physiological dependence?

1. tolerance

2. withdrawal syndrome

13-3   How does the DSM-IV describe substance related disorders?

---

7. a. Substance related disorders are divided into what two subtypes?

1. substance use

2. substance induced

b. What is polysubstance abuse? Abusing several substances at the same time.

8. What is substance abuse? Give an example. drug use resulting recurrent negative social + personal consequences

Example: Can't go to school because of hang over; arrested for drunk driving

9. What is substance dependence? Give an example. *Continued drug use resulting in negative ~~con~~ Consequences + indicators of psychological or psysiological dependence Example: stealing $ to buy drugs; withdrawal symptoms*

13-4   What do we know about alcohol abuse patterns in the United States?

---

10. How have drinking patterns and attitudes about alcohol changed in the last fifteen years? Why have they changed?

11. How would you respond to the following statement? "Twenty years ago, alcohol was a major cause of social problems in the United States. Today, this is no longer true."

12. a.   About what percentage of Americans abstain from alcohol use? *1/3*

    b.   What percentage are light drinkers? *1/3*

    c.   What percentage are moderate to heavy drinkers? *1/3*

13-5   How does alcohol affect the body and behavior?

---

13. In your own words, describe the process that occurs from the time alcohol first enters the stomach until it is metabolized in the liver.

14. a.   If a person is consuming alcohol at a faster rate then the liver can metabolize it, what will happen to the blood alcohol concentration level (BAC)? *it will increase*

b.   What role do the following play on the metabolism of alcohol and the resulting BAC?

1.   eating before drinking *Food in the stomach limits the amount of alcohol transported throughout the blood stream to the brain*

2.   gender *Women metabolize alcohol less effectively than men*

3.   race/ethnic descent *Individuals of asian descent metabolize alcohol more rapidly than most caucasians*

15. Match the following.

1.   _b_   alcoholic cirrhosis
2.   _e_   cardiovascular disease
3.   _a_   pancreatitis
4.   _d_   problems related to immune system suppression
5.   _c_   disorders of the endocrine system

a.   cells in pancreas destroyed

b.   damage to liver cells often seen in men who are heavy drinkers

c.   can lead to problems in sexual behavior and reproduction for both men and women

d.   chronic alcoholics more prone to develop infectious diseases

e.   nondrinkers at slightly higher risk than light or moderate drinkers; heavy drinkers at highest risk to develop several problems

16. a.   What is glutamate? Does alcohol (inhibit) or enhance the activity of glutamate? What effects do you think this would have on brain activity? *Excitatory neurotransmitter. inhibits; dimishes brain cell activity (depressant effect)*

b.   What is GABA? Does alcohol inhibit or (enhance) the activity of GABA? What effects do you think this would have on brain activity? *inhibitor neurotransmitter, enhances activity; dimishes brain cell activity (depressant effect)*

17. a.   Alcohol _____ ((increases) decreases) the level of dopamine in the brain.

Alcohol _____ ((increases) decreases) the level of serotonin in the brain.

Alcohol _____ ((increases) decreases) the level of endogenous opiate endorphins in the brain.

b.   How can the above "reward" the drinker? *Alcohol increases dopamine + serotonin level in "rewards center" of the brain. Alcohol increases release of endogenous opiates which are similar to opiate drugs which produce euphoria + reduce pain.*

18. Fill in the missing information in the table below.

BAC LEVEL	BEHAVIORAL EFFECTS
Below .05	*relaxation; mild loss of inhibitions*
.05 - .08	*slurred speech, mild coordination problems*
.10 and Above	*noticeable coordination problems; mood, drowsiness, perceptual problem, attention*
.25 and Above	*loss of consciousness, death*

19. In your own words, describe how the long-term heavy use of alcohol affects the following.

a.   feelings of agitation and nervousness after drinking *The sedating effect of alcohol wears off before the agitating effects. This causes a rebound effect of agitation after drinking*

b.   tolerance *As tolerance develops due to long-term use, other behavioral effects + personality changes worsen. example: hostility, aggressiveness, brooding*

c.   cognitive functioning *Problem-solving skills, especially those involving ability to concentrate + flexibility in thinking diminish*

13-6   What do we know about the prevalence of alcohol use disorders?

20. Circle the subgroup in each category with the highest rate of alcohol abuse. Underline the group with the lowest rate, if it is listed. *○-highest ___ lowest*

a.   (males)   females

b. (young adults (ages 18 - 29))   any other age group

c. (African American men who drink)   White European American men who drink

d. (African American women who drink)   White European American women who drink

e. (Hispanic American males)   White European American males   Asian Americans
                                                                        (both genders)

| 13-7 | How do we describe patterns of alcohol abuse? |

21. a. In your own words, describe each of Jellineck's four stages of alcohol dependence.

1. prealcoholic phase *occasional social drinking*

2. prodromal phase *heavier (often secret) drink, crucial loss of control when drinking; binging, blackouts, health & social life deteriorates*

3. crucial phase

4. chronic phase *whole life revolves around drinking; malnutrition, physical tolerance; withdrawal symptoms*

b. What are two specific weaknesses of Jellineck's phase model?

1. *Not all alcoholics fit into the different phases*

2. *The model doesn't fit many female alcoholics*

22. Briefly describe characteristics of Type I and Type II alcoholism.

   a. Type I *late onset; prone to anxiety; binge drinking unlikely to behave antisocially when drinking, health problems*

   b. Type II *begins in adolescence; little anxiety; antisocial when drinking, fewer medical problems*

13-8   What other problems are associated with alcohol abuse and dependence?

---

23. Match the following.

   1. __b__ alcohol-induced psychotic disorder
   2. __c__ alcohol induced delirium
   3. __a__ Wernicke-Korsakoff syndrome
   4. __d__ Alcohol induced dementia

   a. caused by alcohol exotoxicity and lack of thiamine

   b. resembles delirium, but often includes hallucinations and delusions

   c. confusion, agitation, inability to attend to the environment

   d. affects memory, language, motor functioning and the ability to plan and organize

24. Respond to the following statement: "It would be productive for researchers to focus on the development of a single factor theory which describes the drinking patterns and problems of all alcoholics. That way, we would be well on our way to understanding the cause of alcoholism."

13-9   What are the possible causes of alcohol use disorders?

---

25. In your own words, briefly describe how each of the following support the view that genetic factors play a role in alcohol abuse? Which, do you feel, are best supported by current research?

   a. family studies *The risk of abuse is 7 times greater among 1st degree relatives of alcoholics than of 1st degree relatives of nonproblem drinkers.*

b.   twin studies   *there is an increase of susceptibility among identical twins than among fraternal twins*

c.   adoption studies   *increase of alcoholics amongst adopted-away children born to alcoholic parents than adopted away children born of non-alcoholic parents*

d.   D2 (dopamine) receptor   *some studies suggest than D2 (dopamine) receptor may be the genic marker for alcoholic vulnerability*

26.   In your own words, briefly describe how each of the following support the view that neurobiological factors play a role in alcohol abuse?

a.   neuroelectrical activity

b.   monoamine oxidase (MAO) and serotonin

c.   heart rate change

27.   In your own words, briefly describe how each of the following support the view that psychological factors play a role in alcohol abuse? Which, do you feel, are best supported by current research?

a.   tension reduction hypothesis

b.   alcohol expectancies

c.   the ability to discern internal cues when drinking

d.   personality (recent studies)

28. In your own words, briefly describe how each of the following support the view that social and cultural factors play a role in alcohol abuse? Which, do you feel, are best supported by current research?

a.   social interaction within the family

b.   peer groups

13-10   How are alcohol use disorders treated?

29. Match the following. (Use some of the alternatives more than once.)

1. __c__ Someone enables the alcoholic to drink, or even prevents positive changes.
2. __b__ More alcoholics are treated by this program than any other.
3. __a__ A four to six week hospital stay is common.
4. __b__ When they feel the need, members go to meetings for support.
5. __a__ "Minnesota model"
6. __b__ 12 steps

   a.   detoxification and inpatient programs

   b.   Alcoholics Anonymous

   c.   family therapy

30. Match the following.

1. __a__ extinction of cues which stimulate alcohol use
2. __b__ used to treat alcohol withdrawal, although some researchers question its use
3. __ed__ useful for problem drinkers who have not developed alcohol dependence

4. _C_ Self deception and faulty decision-making precede return to problem drinking.

5. _b_ There are two approaches: (1) induce unpleasant effects when alcohol is consumed, and (2) block brain functions which cause craving.

6. _d_ One technique is to teach controlled drinking.

7. _a_ Alcoholics learn to reinforce sobriety.

   a.   behavioral treatments

   b.   medication

   c.   relapse prevention programs

   d.   brief intervention

31. In general, why is it important to match different treatment techniques to different types of problem drinkers?

Test your understanding

1. Psychoactive drugs
   a. are substances which affect thinking, emotion and behavior.
   b. are always illegal.
   c. are always harmful to the person.
   d. are always physically and psychologically addictive.

2. Drug use progresses to drug abuse when
   a. the person is using an illegal drug.
   b. the use becomes hazardous to one's health, impairs work or family life, causes personal distress or legal problems.
   c. the person is using more of the drug than most people.
   d. the patterns of drug use fit the DSM-IV criteria for a specific substance use disorder.

3. A pattern in which a person craves a specific drug, is preoccupied with obtaining the substance and continues to consume the drug, even when he or she knows that it is

causing problems is called
   a. polysubstance abuse.
   b. physiological dependence.
   c. withdrawal symptoms.
   d. psychological dependence.

4. Physiological dependence (addiction) is indicated when there is evidence of tolerance and
   a. dementia.
   b. withdrawal.
   c. polydrug use.
   d. delirium.

5. The DSM-IV distinguishes between substance _____ disorders (for example, a student is expelled when marijuana is found in his locker) and substance _____ disorders (for example, physical withdrawal symptoms).
   a. use; induced
   b. induced; use
   c. abuse; intoxication
   d. intoxication; abuse

6. Which of the following statements about alcohol are true?
   a. Alcohol is not a true drug.
   b. Roughly one out of every thirty-three Americans over age eighteen is a moderate to heavy drinker.
   c. African Americans are more likely to abstain from alcohol than are White European Americans.
   d. The percentage of alcohol-related deaths in the United States has steadily increased since 1979.

7. Blood alcohol concentration (BAC)
   a. measures unmetabolized alcohol (ethanol) in the blood.
   b measures metabolized alcohol (ethanol) in the blood.
   c. is a measurement of alcohol (ethanol) in the brain.
   d. is a measurement of alcohol (ethanol) in the stomach.

8. According to Cloninger's model, alcoholics who have a late onset of problem drinking, are prone to anxiety and are unlikely to behave antisocially when drinking, are called
   a. Type I alcoholics.
   b Type II alcoholics.
   c. Type III alcoholics.
   d. Type IV alcoholics.

9. Which of the following statements about Wernicke-Korsakoff syndrome is false?
   a. It is partially caused by a thiamine deficiency.
   b. Confusion and ataxia are often seen in the Wernicke phase.
   c. The loss of memory of general information is seen in the Korsakoff phase.
   d. Persons in the Korsakoff phase tend to confabulate in order to compensate.

10. Adoption studies find that adopted-away children born to alcoholic parents are _____ likely to develop problem drinking in adulthood than adopted-away children born to nonalcoholic parents.
    a. more
    b. less
    c. just as
    d. slightly less

11. Studies attempting to associate biological markers with the potential for alcohol abuse have found differences between alcoholics and nonalcoholics in all of the following except
    a. neuroelectrical activity in the brain.
    b. MAO and serotonin levels.
    c. heart rate levels when drinking.
    d. a prealcoholic gene marker.

12. Which of the following is not associated with the "Minnesota model"?
    a. a strong disease approach
    b. a four to six week hospital stay
    c. detoxification when entering program
    d. each person given an individualized treatment plan, which is based on his or her needs and drinking history

13. Which one of the following does not accurately describe Alcoholics Anonymous?
    a. A.A. offers a 12-step program.
    b. A.A. places a heavy emphasis on alcohol abstinence.
    c. A.A. provides support group meetings.
    d. A.A. provides researchers with a wealth of valuable data and information on alcoholism and alcohol abuse.

14. Relapse prevention programs
    a. are based on the philosophies of A.A.
    b. equate minor isolated relapse with failure.
    c. focus on the drinker's beliefs and decision-making skills.
    d. don't work.

15. Alcohol treatment programs are most effective when
    a.   they are court ordered.
    b.   they are matched to individual variables and needs.
    c.   the patients are Type III alcoholics.
    d.   the alcoholic has "hit bottom."

Answers to test your understanding

1. a.   (13-1)
2. b.   (13-2)
3. d.   (13-2)
4. b.   (13-3)
5. a.   (13-4)
6. c.   (13-4) (13-6)
7. a.   (13-5)
8. a.   (13-7)
9. c.   (13-8)
10. a.   (13-9)
11. d.   (13-9)
12. d.   (13-10)
13. d.   (13-10)
14. c.   (13-10)
15. b.   (13-10)

13-11   What are depressants? How do they affect the body and behavior? How can depressant abuse and dependence be treated?

32. Depressants refer to a group of drugs, including alcohol, that _inhibit_ (increase / inhibit) neurotransmitter activity in the central nervous system. The effects of depressants include sedation, enhanced _sleep_ (anxiety / sleep) and reduced _anxiety_ (anxiety / sleep).

33. Fill in the missing information.

	BARBITURATES Seconal Tuinal phenobarbital	BENZODIAZEPINES Valium Librium Xanax Atavin
Medical Uses	treating anxiety + insomnia	treating auditory + panic disorders, muscle spasms
Effects	relaxation, mild euphoria, impaired motor + cognitive function; depressed blood pressure; depressed respiration	relaxation, euphoria
Health Risks	Coma, death	toxicity + overdose when combined w/ other depressants

34. In your own words, briefly describe the pattern leading to abuse of depressant drugs which are common for each of the following groups.

    a.   adolescents   often recreational + in social settings

b. middle-aged or older middle class *pattern of depressant abuse for middle-age or older middle class persons often begins w/ prescription for anxiety, insomnia + pain.*

c. the elderly *the pattern ~~for~~ of depressant abuse the the elderly often begins w/ prescription for sleep problems. Older persons are more susceptible to the intoxicating effects of the drug + often suffer from memory, cognition, motor*

35. Why is recovery from an addiction to depressant drugs difficult both in detoxification and relapse prevention? *physical withdrawal symptoms ~~complic~~ complicate detoxification; abstinence 3 syndrome complicates relapse prevention*

13-12	What are stimulants? How do they affect the body and behavior? How can stimulant abuse and dependence be treated?

36. Stimulants are a category of drugs which have an _____ ((excitatory) /inhibitory) effect on the central nervous system by _____ (increasing /(decreasing)) the availability of the neurotransmitter _____ ((dopamine) / serotonin).

37. Fill in the missing information in the tables below.

	AMPHETAMINES "speed" Dexedrine Methamphetamine	COCAINE powder "crack"
Medical Uses	*asthma, ADD, obesity, congestion*	*none*
Effects	*alertness, focused attention, aggressiveness, delirium*	*rapid stimulation, euphoria*
Health Risks	*cardiovascular problems, withdrawal dysphoria*	*psychological dependence, respiratory + heart failure, death*

	CAFFEINE coffee tea chocolate	NICOTINE tobacco products
Medical Uses	*cold remedies, diet pills*	none
Effects	*mild stimulation, positive mood, nervousness*	none discussed

agitation, anxiety

Health Risks	*Caffeine intoxication, heart disease*	*Cardiovascular & respiratory disease*

38. Match the following.

1. _d_ nicotine
2. _b_ polydrug use
3. _a_ Cocaine Anonymous
4. _C_ Azrin's community reinforcement model
5. _e_ node-link mapping
6. _f_ using medication to treat stimulant abuse

a. a 12-step program used to help prevent relapse

b. often develops in an attempt to "take the edge off" and complicates treatment

c. treatment approach which reinforces cocaine abstinence, may be superior to 12-step programs

d. commonly used drug, but is a deadly poison in its pure form

e. representation of thoughts, feelings and actions that precede and follow cocaine use

f. limited success in counteracting the effects of stimulants and the withdrawal symptoms

---

13-13 What are opiates? How do they affect the body and behavior? How can opiate abuse and dependence be treated?

---

39. Opiates, also known as _____ (narcotics / stimulants), affect the user by interacting with the body's _____ (endogenous / exogenous) opiates, including endorphins and enkephalins.

40. In your own words, explain the probable cause of opiate withdrawal symptoms, especially those of negative mood and increased pain sensitivity.

Both endogenous (natural) opiates & exogenous opiates (morphine = example) influence pain sensitivity & positive mood. When exogenous opiates are frequently ingested, endogenous opiates production is slowed. If the intake of exogenous opiates is stopped, low levels of both will result in + both mood & pain sensitivity will be affected.

41. Fill in the missing information.

OPIATES (NARCOTICS)		
morphine heroin codeine methadone		
Medical Uses	*Pain reduction*	

Effects	*dulled senses + attention, dream-like euphoria, depression, coma*
Health Risks	*~~help~~ respiratory failure, intense withdrawal symptoms, death*

42. a. In your own words, describe the positive aspects of methadone maintenance therapy as a treatment for heroin addiction. *MMT may ~~help~~ reduce illicit opiate use, criminal activity + the transmission of infectious diseases). Addicts stay in treatment longer*

b. In your own words, describe the negative aspects with methadone maintenance therapy as a treatment for heroin addiction. *addicts remain dependent these programs may ~~also~~ actually increase inappropriate drug use*

c. Many experts believe that methadone maintenance programs are _____ (more / less) effective when paired with psychological treatments.

13-14	What are the effects of cannabis and hallucinogens? How are they abused and how are problems associated with these substances treated?

43. Fill in the missing information in the table below.

	CANNABIS (THC) marijuana hashish	HALLUCINOGENS LSD mescaline PCP psilocybin MDMA
Medical Uses	*anorexia, glaucoma, nausea*	*none*
Effects	*mild euphoria mild perceptual distortions*	*variable mood, ~~the~~ perceptual distortions, depersonalization, paranoid thinking, synesthesia*
Health Risks	*variable mood per-ceptual distortions, depersonalization, paranoid thinking, synesthesia*	*flashbacks, panic attacks (LSD), fatal overdose (PCP)*

44. Match the following.

1. _a_ cannabis (*marijuana*)
2. _b_ synesthesia

3.   _c_ LSD
4.   _d_ phencyclidine (PCP)

   a.   amotivational syndrome

   b.   a perceptual distortion common with hallucinogen use

   c.   strong hallucinogen popular in the 1960's and 1970's whose use declined, but now seems to be increasing

   d.   overdose of this hallucinogen can be fatal

Test your understanding

1.   In general, depressant drugs reduce activity in the brain and nervous system by enhancing the activity of
   a.   serotonin.
   b.   dopamine.
   c.   GABA.
   d.   opiates.

2.   The chance of overdosing on depressants increases dramatically when
   a.   the person has not developed a physical tolerance for the drug.
   b.   the depressant is taken in combination with stimulant drugs.
   c.   the depressant is taken in combination with other depressant drugs.
   d.   the person taking the drug is tired, depressed or under a significant amount of stress.

3.   In general, stimulant drugs have an excitatory effect on the brain and nervous system by increasing the activity of
   a.   serotonin.
   b.   dopamine.
   c.   endogenous opiates.
   d.   monoamine oxidase.

4.   The effects of cocaine differ from amphetamines in that
   a.   cocaine produces a less euphoric experience than do amphetamines.
   b.   cocaine produces more rapid, but shorter lasting effects than do amphetamines.
   c.   the behavioral effects of the two are about the same; the physiological effects are different.
   d.   cocaine intoxication lasts up to twice as long as amphetamine intoxication.

5.   Stimulant users are prone to _____ in an attempt to "take the edge off."
   a.   drop out of treatment
   b.   abuse more and more stimulants
   c.   polydrug use
   d.   denial

6.   Node-link mapping is
   a.   a method used in conducting urine tests for ex-addicts.
   b.   a process where drug users construct charts which depict personal issues and behavior patterns which are associated with their drug use.
   c.   step 4 in most 12 step programs.
   d.   a method for keeping track of the different substances abused by polydrug users.

7. In its pure form nicotine is
    a.   harmless.
    b.   similar in chemical makeup to THC.
    c.   a deadly poison.
    d.   not a drug.

8. One year following completion of stop smoking programs, cigarette abstinence rates rarely exceed
    a.   10 percent.
    b.   30 percent.
    c.   50 percent.
    d.   75 percent.

9. Withdrawal from opiates often includes symptoms of negative mood and increased pain sensitivity. This is because
    a.   exogenous opiates, such as heroin, use the same receptor sites as endogenous opiates.
    b.   there is a synergetic effect between various types of opiate drugs.
    c.   opiates, such as morphine, decrease dopamine activity in the brain.
    d.   opiates, such as morphine, decrease serotonin levels in the brain.

10. Methadone is a
    a.   famous treatment center for drug addicts in New York City.
    b.   neurotransmitter affected by opiates.
    c.   drug used to treat cocaine abuse.
    d.   synthetic opiate used in the treatment of opiate abuse.

11. Which one of the following statements about cannabis is false?
    a.   The main active ingredient of cannabis is THC.
    b.   Cannabis is the most commonly used illicit drug in the United States.
    c.   Tolerance and withdrawal are not prominent problems associated with the use of cannabis.
    d.   Research confirms that chronic use of cannabis directly causes amotivational syndrome.

12. Cannabis use among young people
    a.   has been decreasing steadily for the last twenty years.
    b.   had been declining, but recently has increased in popularity.
    c.   has remained steady over the last 20 years.
    d.   has all but disappeared.

13. Which one of the following statements about hallucinogens is false?
    a.   Hallucinogens can cause synesthesia.
    b.   Hallucinogens affect perception, but not mood.
    c.   Hallucinogens can cause depersonalization, paranoid thinking and distorted body image.
    d.   The effects of hallucinogens can last from a few hours or as long as a day.

14. LSD has been used to study the neurological processes associated with
    a.   schizophrenia.
    b.   dissociative disorders.
    c.   mental retardation.
    d.   depression.

15. Which of the following statements about PCP is false?
    a   PCP is more popular than LSD in poor urban neighborhoods.
    b.   Unlike the other hallucinogens, PCP does not produce hallucinations or perceptual distortions.
    c.   PCP often produces violent reactions.
    d.   Unlike the other hallucinogens, PCP overdoses can be fatal.

Answers to test your understanding

1.   c.   (13-11)
2.   c.   (13-11)
3.   b.   (13-12)
4.   b.   (13-12)
5.   c.   (13-12)
6.   b.   (13-12)
7.   c.   (13-12)
8.   c.   (13-12)
9.   a.   (13-13)
10.   d.   (13-13)
11.   d.   (13-14)
12.   b.   (13-14)
13.   b.   (13-14)
14.   a.   (13-14)
15.   b.   (13-14)

When you have finished . . .

Explore the Web to find more information

The National Clearinghouse for Alcohol and Drug Information is a good place to start if you're looking for general material on substance abuse issues. You can find resources and referral information, as well as informational and statistical databases. The Clearinghouse is a service of **The Center for Substance Abuse Prevention**, **The Substance Abuse and Mental Health Services Administration**, the **U.S. Public Health Service** and the **U.S. Department of Health and Human Services**. You will find the site at (**http://www.health.org/**).

The Boston University Medical Center Community Outreach Health Information System provides information on most of the drugs discussed in this chapter. Their Alcohol and Substance Abuse Page can be accessed at (**http://web.bu.edu/COHIS/subsabse/subsabse.htm**).

Information on second-hand smoke is available from the **Center For Health Statistics**, which is associated with the **Centers For Disease Control**. (**http://www.cdc.gov/nchswww/releases/nrsmoke.htm**)

An informative document from **The American Academy of Child and Adolescent Psychiatry** titled, "Making Decisions About Substance Abuse Treatment," can be accessed at (**http://www.psych.med.umich.edu/web/aacap/factsFam/subabuse.htm**).

At the **Alcoholics Anonymous** Web site (**http://www.alcoholics-anonymous.org /**) you will find an A.A. fact file as well as other A.A. related information.

Cocaine Anonymous (**http://www.ca.org/index.html**). Here you will find an interesting self-test for cocaine addiction as well as referral phone numbers.

The Youth to Youth Teen Peer Prevention Program from South Kingstown High School, Wakefield, RI. (**http://198.115.232.254/Y2Y/**), is a wonderful example of a teen drug prevention program. Their Web site includes quite a bit of drug information as well as numerous links to other sites.

As you read in this chapter, there is disagreement among clinicians as to the value of methadone maintenance treatment programs. For one view, go to the **National Alliance of Methadone Advocates** site at (**http://methadone.org/**). NAMA is an organization composed of methadone maintenance patients and supporters who are committed to "promoting quality methadone maintenance treatment as the most effective modality for the treatment of heroin addiction." Some of the many links at this site include:

    The Origin of Methadone Maintenance
    How Methadone Works
    The Discovery of Endorphin
    Test Your Knowledge About Methadone Maintenance

After you investigate this Web site, see if you can track down information presented by representatives of the opposing view.

CHAPTER 14
Sexual and Gender Identity Disorders

Before you read . . .

Survey the chapter

Chapter 14 begins with the case of John, a 28-year-old postal employee who, since childhood, has always thought of himself as a woman trapped in a man's body. The realities of situations such as John's pose questions which will be addressed in this chapter. Does John have a mental disorder? What factors bring about such variations in sexual expression? Can, or should, John receive treatment to accept his maleness?

Chapter 14 focuses on three types of sexual and gender identity disorders: gender identity disorders which are characterized by a person's dissatisfaction with his or her biological gender; sexual dysfunction, in which a person's ability to function sexually is limited or disturbed; and paraphilias, which involve sexual arousal that is repeatedly elicited by inanimate objects or other inappropriate stimuli or situations.

As you read . . .

Ask questions

14-1   What is the difference between gender identity, sex roles, sexual orientation and sexual behavior?

14-2   How have researchers studied the various patterns of human sexual behavior and what have they learned?

14-3   What biological factors influence the physical aspects of human sexual differences?

14-4   Are variations in sexual orientation, such as homosexuality, classified as mental disorders?

14-5   How common are variations in sexual orientation?

14-6   What biological and psychological factors influence sexual orientation?

14-7   What are gender identity disorders?

14-8   What causes gender identity disorders?

14-9   How are gender identity disorders treated?

14-10   What are sexual dysfunction disorders?

14-11   What factors influence sexual responsiveness?

14-12   What are the characteristics of sexual desire disorders?

14-13   What are the characteristics of sexual arousal disorders?

14-14   What are the characteristics of orgasmic disorders?

14-15   What are the characteristics of sexual pain disorders?

14-16   How are sexual dysfunction disorders treated?

14-17   What is paraphilia and what forms can it take?

14-18   What are the causes of paraphilias?

14-19   Can paraphilias be effectively treated?

After you read . . .

Review and explore the chapter

14-1   What is the difference between gender identity, sex roles, sexual orientation and sexual behavior?

1.   Match the following.

   1.   ____ gender identity
   2.   ____ cross-gender identification
   3.   ____ gender or sex role
   4.   ____ sexual orientation
   5.   ____ homosexual behavior
   6.   ____ heterosexual behavior
   7.   ____ bisexual behavior

    a.   a person's tendency or preference for engaging in sexual behavior with male or female partners

    b.   patterns of behavior typically expected of males or females in a particular culture

    c.   sexual activity with members of the opposite sex

    d.   sexual activity with members of the same sex

    e.   preoccupation with the desire to live as the other sex

    f.   sexual activity with members of both sexes

    g.   a person's sense of being male or female

2.   Are gender identity, sex roles, sexual orientation and sexual behavior independent of each other or are these different aspects of sexuality locked together in specific patterns?

14-2   How have researchers studied the various patterns of human sexual behavior and what have they learned?

---

3.   One of the first large-scale surveys of sexual behavior in the United states was conducted by _____ (Alfred Kinsey / Playboy Magazine). The results of this survey, as with others, have been viewed with some skepticism because the people studied may not have been _____ (honest about / representative of) the adult population about which conclusions have been drawn. The latest, most representative and scientifically constructed survey is the _____ (National Health and Social Life Survey / The Hite Report).

4.   a.   Is the study of sexual fantasies a legitimate method for investigation of sexuality?

    b.   Do men or women fantasize more about sex?

    c.   According to one study, what is the most common sexual fantasy for both men and women?

14-3   What biological factors influence the physical aspects of human sexual differences?

5.   In your own words, briefly describe the biological processes affecting the physical aspects of sexual differences which occur at each of the following stages of life.

a.   conception -- the X and Y chromosomes

b.   eight to twelve weeks after conception

c.   puberty

6.   a.   What is congenital adrenal hyperplasis?

b.   What is testicular feminization?

14-4   Are variations in sexual orientation, such as homosexuality, classified as mental disorders?

7.   How has homosexuality been classified by the American Psychiatric Association

a.   before 1973 (DSM-I and early DSM-II)?

b.   from 1973-1979 (late DSM-II)?

c.   from 1980-1986 (DSM-III)?

d.   from 1987-present (DSM-III-R and DSM-IV)?

8.   As a group, homosexuals have been perceived historically as not psychologically well adjusted. Is this an accurate view?

14-5   How common are variations in sexual orientation?

9.   Homosexual orientations are found in _____ (few / most) societies. In one study, _____ (less than 10 / over 60) percent of non-Western cultures included homosexual activities as an acceptable form of sexual behavior. From the information gathered in Kinsey's original survey, many concluded that approximately _____ (1 percent / 10 percent) of Americans are homosexual. However, more recent studies suggest that this figure may be somewhat _____ (low / high).

14-6   What biological and psychological factors influence sexual orientation?

10.   In your own words, briefly describe how research in each of the following areas may point to a relationship between biological factors and homosexuality.

a.   twin studies

b.   the X chromosome

c.   neuroanatomy

    d.   prenatal hormones

    e.   birth order and sibling gender

11. a.   Have any well-controlled studies been able to confirm a clear role for psychological factors in homosexuality?

    b.   Does growing up in a family with a homosexual parent make it more likely that a child will become homosexual?

14-7   What are gender identity disorders?

12. Gender identity disorders involve confusion or dissatisfaction with one's biological gender. These disorders always involve two components. What are they?

    a.

    b.

13. a.   What term is often applied to adults who experience gender identity disorder?

    b.   How does this term differ from the term, hermaphrodite?

14. a.   Are gender identity disorders more often diagnosed in boys or girls? Why?

   b.   Are gender identity disorders more prevalent in children or adults? Why?

15. Use the table below to describe the common characteristics or typical behaviors seen in children with gender identity disorder at different ages.

TIME PERIOD	COMMON CHARACTERISTICS / TYPICAL BEHAVIORS
Infancy	
Ages two to three	
Kindergarten	
School aged	

16. For most people, do gender identity disorders which present in childhood persist into adulthood?

17. Adult transsexuals fall into two categories. What are they?

   a.

   b.

14-8   What causes gender identity disorders?

---

18. Have researchers been able to establish a link between genetics and gender identity disorders?

19. Could parenting practices and expectations be responsible for gender identity disorders?

14-9   How are gender identity disorders treated?

---

20. In your own words, briefly describe the most common psychological interventions used to alter gender identity.

21. In your own words, briefly describe sex reassignment surgery.

Test your understanding

1. A person's sense of being male or female is called
    a.   gender identity.
    b.   cross-gender identity.
    c.   gender role or sex role.
    d.   sexual orientation.

2. A person's tendency or preference for engaging in sexual behavior with male or female partners is called
    a.   gender identity.
    b.   cross-gender identity.
    c.   gender role or sex role.
    d.   sexual orientation.

3. One of the first large-scale surveys of sexual behavior in the United States was done by
    a.   Masters and Johnson.
    b.   Alfred Kinsey.
    c.   Sigmund Freud.
    d.   the University of Denver.

4. A fetus has received one X and one Y chromosome. Six weeks after conception
    a.   the fetus is easily recognizable as a male.
    b.   the fetus is easily recognizable as a female.
    c.   it would be impossible to determine sex, as males and females develop exactly the same for the first eight to twelve weeks. In time however, male

genitalia will develop.

d.   it would be impossible to determine sex, as males and females develop exactly the same for the first eight to twelve weeks. In time however, female genitalia will develop.

5.   What is testicular feminization?

a.   an early form of male-to-female sex reassignment surgery

b.   a new and relatively simple procedure which takes the place of dangerous and expensive male-to-female sex reassignment surgery

c.   a genetic defect on the Y chromosome which causes males to be born with female genitalia

d.   a rite of passage performed on males in various cultures

6.   How have the various editions of the DSM classified homosexuality?

a.   Prior to 1973, it was listed as a mental disorder. Today, it is not.

b.   Prior to 1973, it was not listed as a mental disorder. Today, it is.

c.   Homosexuality has been classified as a mental disorder in every edition of the DSM.

d.   Homosexuality has never been classified as a mental disorder in any edition of the DSM.

7.   As a group, homosexuals have often been perceived as not psychologically well adjusted. Is this an accurate view?

a.   Yes, studies have consistently shown that although the rates of mental illness in most categories are equivalent for homosexuals and heterosexuals, homosexuals display a much higher rate of paraphilia and fetish disorders.

b.   Yes, studies have consistently shown that although the rates of mental illness in most categories are equivalent for homosexuals and heterosexuals, homosexuals display a much higher

rate of personality disorders.

c.   Yes, studies have consistently shown that although the rates of mental illness in most categories are equivalent for homosexuals and heterosexuals, homosexuals tend to function much less adequately in their daily lives.

d.   No, studies have revealed no significant differences in the prevalence of mental disorders or the overall quality of functioning between homosexuals and heterosexuals.

8.   Homosexual orientations have been found

a.   in very few societies.

b.   in about half of the societies studied.

c.   in most societies.

d.   only in urbanized, Western cultures.

9.   Which figure below is probably closest to the actual prevalence rate of homosexuality in the United States?

a.   less than 1 percent

b.   4-10 percent

c.   15-18 percent

d.   above 20 percent

10.   Which of the following is probably the most accurate statement about the causes of homosexuality?

a.   The development of a homosexual orientation is most influenced by interaction with homosexuals before the age of two.

b.   The development of a homosexual orientation is most influenced by interaction with homosexuals when the person is at or slightly before puberty.

c.   The development of a homosexual orientation is most influenced by the lack of a strong gender role model, especially before age five.

d.   Homosexual orientation is shaped by one or more biological factors, including genetics, neuroanatomical differences or hormonal influences.

11. Which of the following statements about gender identity disorders is not true?
     a.   One component of gender identity disorders is persistent cross-gender identification.
     b.   One component of gender identity disorders is profound discomfort or even disgust with one's biological sex and sexual organs.
     c.   Children who experience gender identity disorders are sometimes termed hermaphrodites.
     d.   Adults who experience gender identity disorders are sometimes termed transsexuals.

12. Which of the following statements about gender identity disorders is not true?
     a.   Gender identity disorders are diagnosed more often in boys.
     b.   Gender identity disorders are diagnosed more often in children than adults.
     c.   If gender identity disorders are experienced in childhood, they will often persist into adulthood.
     d.   Gender identity disorders usually begin to develop at a very early age.

13. Adult transsexuals
     a.   are exclusively homosexual in orientation.
     b.   are exclusively bisexual in orientation.
     c.   are exclusively heterosexual in orientation.
     d.   may be either homosexual, bisexual or heterosexual in orientation.

14. The major causal factors in the development of gender identity disorders
     a.   are unknown.
     b.   are genetic.
     c.   are related to brain structure and chemistry.
     d.   are psychological.

15. All of the following are common methods used in the treatment of gender identity disorders except
     a.   sex reassignment surgery for adults.
     b.   electroconvulsive shock therapy (ECT) for adults.
     c.   behavior therapy for children, such as modeling and reinforcing gender appropriate behaviors.
     d.   coaching parents about how to reshape their child's behavior.

Answers to test your understanding

1.   a.   (14-1)
2.   d.   (14-1)
3.   b.   (14-2)
4.   c.   (14-3)
5.   c.   (14-3)
6.   a.   (14-4)
7.   d.   (14-4)
8.   c.   (14-5)
9.   b.   (14-5)
10. d.   (14-6)
11. c.   (14-7)
12. c.   (14-7)
13. d.   (14-7)
14. a.   (14-8)
15. b.   (14-9)

14-10   What are sexual dysfunction disorders?

22. Sexual dysfunction disorders involve pain associated with sexual intercourse and/or problems with the fist three phases of the sexual response cycle. In your own words, briefly describe each of the stages of the sexual response cycle.

    a.   desire phase

    b.   excitement phase

    c.   orgasmic phase

    d.   resolution phase

23. Who were William Masters and Virginia Johnson? What effect did they have on our understanding of sexual response cycle and the theory and treatment of sexual dysfunction?

14-11   What factors influence sexual responsiveness?

24. In your own words, briefly describe how each of the following affect sexual responsiveness.

    a.   neurological and vascular factors

    b.   attitudes and beliefs

c.   interpersonal factors

14-12   What are the characteristics of sexual desire disorders?

25. Fill in the missing information about hypoactive sexual desire disorder in the table below.

HYPOACTIVE SEXUAL DESIRE DISORDER (HSDD)		
Typical Characteristics		
Prevalence		
Possible Biological Causes	Men	
	Women	
Possible Psychological Causes	Early Childhood	
	Other	

26. What is sexual aversion disorder?

14-13   What are the characteristics of sexual arousal disorders?

27. Fill in the missing information about sexual arousal disorders in the table below.

SEXUAL AROUSAL DISORDERS		
	FEMALE SEXUAL AROUSAL DISORDER	MALE ERECTILE DISORDER
Typical Features		
Prevalence	no information	
Possible Biological Causes		

Possible Psychological Causes		

14-14   What are the characteristics of orgasmic disorders?

28. Fill in the missing information about orgasmic disorders in the table below.

ORGASMIC DISORDERS			
	FEMALE ORGASMIC DISORDER	MALE ORGASMIC DISORDER	PREMATURE EJACULATION
Typical Features			
Prevalence			
Possible Biological Causes			
Possible Psychological Causes			

14-15   What are the characteristics of sexual pain disorders?

29.

SEXUAL PAIN DISORDERS		
	DYSPAREUNIA	VAGINISMUS
Typical Features		
Prevalence		
Possible Biological Causes		
Possible Psychological Causes		

14-16   How are sexual dysfunction disorders treated?

30. In your own words, briefly describe the treatment model used by Masters and Johnson. Don't forget to discuss the use of sensate focus in your answer.

31. a.   Are disorders of sexual desire more or less difficult to treat than problems of arousal or orgasm?

    b.   Briefly discuss four approaches for treating problems of arousal and orgasm.

        1.

        2.

        3.

        4.

32. Fill in the missing information in the table below.

	SPECIFIC TREATMENT TECHNIQUES
Female Sexual Arousal Disorder	
Male Erectile Disorder	

Female Orgasmic Disorder	
Premature Ejaculation	
Sexual Pain Disorders	

14-17   What is paraphilia and what forms can it take?

33. What is the main feature of all types of paraphilia?

34. Match the following.

1. fetishism
2. transsexual fetishism
3. exhibitionism
4. voyeurism
5. frotteurism
6. sexual masochism
7. sexual sadism
8. pedophilia

a. involves recurrent touching or rubbing against a nonconsenting person in order to become aroused or sexually gratified

b. sexual arousal or gratification depends on receiving painful stimulation or being humiliated

c. sexual arousal and satisfaction through the clandestine observation of others undressing or engaging in sexual activity

d. obtaining sexual arousal or gratification by inflicting painful stimulation or by humiliating one's sexual partner

e. male cross-dressing for sexual arousal and satisfaction

f. recurrent and highly arousing fantasias, urges or behaviors involving a prepubescent child, by a person over age sixteen and at least five years older than the child

g. sexual arousal and satisfaction necessitates the use of an inanimate object

      h.   sexual excitement and satisfaction from the act of exposing one's genitals to an unwilling observer

35. a.   Why is rape not categorized as a paraphilia?

      b.   In your own words, briefly describe four subtypes of rapists.

         1.

         2.

         3.

         4.

14-18   What are the causes of paraphilias?

36. Do biological factors such as genetics seem to be related to the development of paraphilias?

37. In your own words, briefly describe three psychological theories which attempt to explain the development of paraphilias.

    a.

    b.

c.

14-19   Can paraphilias be effectively treated?

---

38. Describe how behavior therapy is sometimes used to treat paraphilias.

39. Describe how multimodal treatment is sometimes used with paraphilias.

Test your understanding

1. Which of the following lists all of the phases of the human sexual response in their correct order.
   a. desire - orgasmic - excitement - resolution
   b. desire - excitement - orgasmic - resolution
   c. excitement - orgasmic - resolution - increased desire
   d. excitement - desire - orgasmic - resolution

2. The researchers who, beginning in the late 1950's, conducted landmark studies detailing the physiological aspects of the human sexual response and sexual dysfunction were
   a. Alfred Kinsey and associates.
   b. Masters and Johnson.
   c. Torvil and Dean.
   d. associated with the University of Illinois and funded by Playboy magazine.

3. Can sexual responsiveness be affected by neurological and vascular factors, attitudes and beliefs and interpersonal relationships?
   a. Yes, all three play a vital role in sexual responsiveness.
   b. No, sexual responsiveness is biological in nature, therefore, only neurological and vascular factors are important.
   c. No, sexual responsiveness is psychological in nature, therefore, only attitudes and beliefs are important.
   d. No, sexual responsiveness is social in nature, therefore, only the quality of the interpersonal relationship is important.

4. Infrequent interest or motivation for sexual activity which causes distress and/or relationship problems is called
   a. sexual aversion disorder (SAD).
   b. nonresponsive sexual dysfunction disorder (NSDD).
   c. hypoactive sexual desire disorder (HSDD).
   d. impotence in males, frigidity in females.

5. Which of the following statements about sexual arousal disorders is not true?
   a. Female sexual arousal disorder involves distressing, persistent problems in attaining or maintaining lubrication and genital swelling during sexual activity.
   b. Female sexual arousal disorder is sometimes related to childhood abuse.
   c. Male erectile disorder involves distressing, persistent failure to attain or maintain an erection adequate for sexual activity.
   d. Male erectile disorder is quite rare in healthy men.

6. Which of the following is not a common orgasmic disorder?
   a. female orgasmic disorder
   b. male orgasmic disorder
   c. premature ejaculation
   d. male erectile disorder

7. Which of the following statements about sexual pain disorders is not true?
   a. Dyspareunia involves recurring problems with pain before, during or after sexual intercourse.
   b. Vaginismus involves involuntary muscle spasms of the vagina, which make penetration impossible.
   c. As with vaginismus, dyspareunia occurs only in women.
   d. The prevalence of vaginismus varies from culture to culture, with rates being higher in places with restrictive attitudes about sexuality.

8. Which of the following intervention techniques for the treatment of sexual dysfunction is most closely associated with Masters and Johnson?
   a. sensate focus
   b. medication
   c. parental coaching and modeling
   d. touch and go

9. Which of the following statements about disorders of sexual desire is false?
   a. Disorders of sexual desire are often treated with cognitive-behavioral techniques.
   b. Disorders of sexual desire are sometimes treated by using sexual scripts.
   c. Disorders of sexual desire are sometimes treated with medication.
   d. Disorders of sexual desire are generally easier to treat than are problems of arousal and orgasm.

10. A client seeking treatment for a sexual problem has been told that the squeeze technique, stop-and-start technique, anxiety reduction and possibly medication may be of use. The problem which the client is seeking help for is probably
    a. female orgasmic disorder.
    b. premature ejaculation.
    c. male erectile disorder.
    d. female sexual arousal disorder.

11. Which of the paraphilias involves recurrent touching or rubbing against a nonconsenting person in order to become aroused or sexually gratified?
    a. fetishism
    b. voyeurism
    c. frotteurism
    d. pedophilia

12. In which of the paraphilias does sexual arousal and satisfaction necessitate the use of an inanimate object?
    a. fetishism
    b. voyeurism
    c. frotteurism
    d. pedophilia

13. Is rape classified as a paraphilia?
    a. Yes.
    b. Yes, but only in cases involving pedophilia.
    c. No, because rape is a crime of

violence, not a sexual disorder.

d.   No, because rape is classified as an
     Axis II disorder.

14. Which of the following has the least support
     as a possible contributing factor for
     paraphilias?
     a.   genetics
     b.   sexual stressors in childhood
     c.   classical conditioning
     d.   the influence of popular media and
          social values

15. Which therapy below has historically been a
     popular method for the treatment of
     paraphilias?
     a.   electroconvulsive shock therapy (ECT)
     b.   behavior therapy, especially aversion
          therapy
     c.   traditional psychoanalytic therapy
     d.   psychosurgery

Answers to test your understanding

1. b.   (14-10)
2. b.   (14-10)
3. a.   (14-11)
4. c.   (14-12)
5. d.   (14-13)
6. d.   (14-14)
7. c.   (14-15)
8. a.   (14-16)
9. d.   (14-16)
10. b.   (14-16)
11. c.   (14-17)
12. a.   (14-17)
13. c.   (14-17)
14. a.   (14-18)
15. b.   (14-19)

When you have finished . . .

Explore the Web to find more information

The **American Psychological Association** provides the document, "Answers to Your Questions About Sexual Orientation and Homosexuality," at (**http://www.apa.org/pubinfo/orient.html**).

Internet Mental Health provides an article on sexual orientation by John Money, Ph.D.   The article, "The Development of Sexual Orientation," was published in the Harvard Medical School Mental Health Letter, February, 1988 and can be accessed at (**http://www.mentalhealth.com/mag1/p5h-sx01.html**).

In 1992, the **National Institutes of Health Consensus Development Conference on Impotence** "was convened to address (1) the prevalence and clinical, psychological and social impact of erectile dysfunction; (2) the risk factors for erectile dysfunction and how they might be used in preventing its development; (3) the need for and appropriate diagnostic assessment and evaluation of patients with erectile dysfunction; (4) the efficacies and risks of behavioral, pharmacological, surgical and other treatments for erectile dysfunction; (5) strategies for improving public and professional awareness and knowledge of erectile dysfunction; and (6) future directions for research in prevention, diagnosis and management of erectile dysfunction. Following 2 days of presentations by experts and discussion by the audience, a consensus panel weighed the evidence and prepared their consensus statement." The complete text of that statement is available at (**http://text.nlm.nih.gov/nih/cdc/www/91txt.html#Head14**).

Another very in depth discussion of erectile dysfunction is available through **The National Institute of Diabetes and Digestive and Kidney Diseases of the National Institutes of Health**. You will find this at (**http://www.niddk.nih.gov/Impotence/Impotnce.html**).

A number of links dealing with endometriosis are provided by **CliniWeb**, sponsored by **Oregon Health Sciences University** and **The National Library of Medicine**. You will find it by going to (**http://www.ohsu.edu/cliniweb/C13/C13.371.html**).

CHAPTER 15
Biological Treatment of Mental Disorders

Before you read . . .

Survey the chapter

Chapter 15 discusses the three main forms of biological treatment of mental disorders. The first, psychosurgery, goes back to prehistoric times when holes were drilled in the skull in an attempt to release evil spirits. This gave way to an era of imprecise and often destructive lobotomies. Finally, today's modern surgical techniques were developed.

The second biological treatment is electroconvulsive therapy. As you will see, after harsh beginnings, this form of treatment has evolved into an humane and legitimate therapeutic intervention.

The last biologically-based therapy discussed is the use of psychoactive medications, a form of treatment which has grown dramatically in the last fifty years. The general categories of commonly used medications, their effects, as well as possible side effects and guidelines for use are discussed.

As you read . . .

Ask questions

15-1   What kinds of psychosurgery have been used in the past?

15-2   How is psychosurgery used today?

15-3   What types of convulsive therapy have been tried in the past?

15-4   What is electroconvulsive therapy?

15-5   Why is the use of psychoactive drug therapy increasing in popularity?

15-6   How do psychoactive drugs work?

15-7   What medications are commonly used to treat mood disorders? How do they work?

15-8   What medications are commonly used in the treatment of anxiety disorders? How do they work?

15-9   What medications are commonly used in the treatment of schizophrenia? How do they work?

15-10   What medications are commonly used in the treatment of attention-deficit/hyperactivity disorder? How do they work?

15-11   How do ethnicity and gender relate to psychoactive drugs?

After you read . . .

Review and explore the chapter

15-1   What kinds of psychosurgery have been used in the past?

1.   What was trephining? When was it used?

2.   Match the following.

1.   ____ Antonio de Egas Moniz
2.   ____ Walter Freeman and James Watts
3.   ____ prefrontal leucotomy (lobotomy)
4.   ____ standard lobotomy (frontal lobotomy)
5.   ____ transorbital lobotomy
6.   ____ "blind" psychosurgery

 a.   true of early procedures, surgeon unsure of exactly what areas of the brain were being lesioned

 b.   a cutting instrument was inserted through holes drilled in the side of the skull and then pivoted, severing connections between the frontal lobes and the rest of the brain

 c.   introduced prefrontal leucotomy, received Nobel prize for medicine in 1949

 d.   instrument similar to an ice pick inserted into the eye socket and tapped into frontal lobes

 e.   developed standard and transorbital lobotomies

 f.   the first of the lobotomy procedures, alcohol inserted into holes in skull to destroy tissue in frontal lobes; later, an instrument was used

3.   What were some of the side effects from "blind" surgical procedures?

| 15-2 | How is psychosurgery used today? |

4.   What is the major difference between modern psychosurgical procedures and the "blind" procedures of the past?

5.   What is the most common psychosurgery procedure done in North America today? Describe how it is done, why it is done and possible side effects.

6.   Describe stereotaxic subcaudate tractotomy (SST).

7.   Patients with what type of mental disorders are most likely to benefit from psychosurgery?

8.   What are four reasons why it is difficult to assess the effectiveness of psychosurgery?

     a.

     b.

     c.

d.

15-3   What types of convulsive therapy have been tried in the past?

9.   In your own words, briefly describe Sakel's use of insulin coma as therapy. Did it prove to be effective?

10. In your own words, briefly describe Meduna's use of metrazol induced seizures as therapy. Did it prove to be effective?

15-4   What is electroconvulsive therapy?

11. a.   In your own words, briefly describe Cerletti and Bini's use of electroconvulsive shock therapy (ECT).

     b.   In what ways has modern ECT been refined in order to minimize the serious side effects which were common with Cerletti and Bini's original procedure?

     c.   What are the common side effects of modern ECT?

12. Which kinds of mental disorders are treated with ECT today? Is this treatment effective?

13. In your own words, briefly describe two prominent theories which attempt to explain the therapeutic effects of ECT.

a.

b.

Test your understanding

1. Drilling holes in the skull in order to allow the cause of the behavioral problem to escape is called
   a. trephining.
   b. transorbital lobotomy.
   c. cingulotomy.
   d. ECT.

2. An instrument similar to an ice pick is inserted above the eyeball and tapped into the frontal lobes of the brain. This describes
   a. trephining.
   b. transorbital lobotomy.
   c. cingulotomy.
   d. ECT.

3. Who were Walter Freeman and James Watts?
   a. They were physicians who developed the first prefrontal leucotomy.
   b. They were physicians who developed the standard and transorbital lobotomies.
   c. They were politicians who lead the fight to ban the use of lobotomy.
   d. They were psychologists who lead the fight to ban the use of all psychosurgery.

4. What is the most common psychosurgery done in North America today?
   a. trephining
   b. transorbital lobotomy
   c. cingulotomy
   d. ECT

5. Patients with what type of mental disorders are most likely to benefit from psychosurgery?
   a. certain types of schizophrenia
   b. somatoform and dissociative disorders that do not respond to drugs or other treatment
   c. delirium and dementia that do not respond to drugs or other treatment
   d. severe depression and bipolar disorder, and extreme cases of OCD that do not respond to drugs or other treatment

6. In the 1930's Viennese psychiatrist, Manfred Sakel
   a. developed and promoted insulin coma therapy.
   b. developed and promoted metrazol induced seizures as therapy.
   c. developed and promoted electroconvulsive shock therapy.
   d. lead the fight to ban convulsive therapies.

7. Metrazol induced seizure therapy
    a. has proven to be effective for treating schizophrenia.
    b. is used today more than electroconvulsive therapy, because there are fewer negative side effects.
    c. is no longer used, because it is not effective.
    d. is no longer used, because it is too expensive.

8. Who first developed and promoted ECT?
    a. Masters and Johnson
    b. Cerletti and Bini
    c. Metrazol and Meduna
    d. Freeman and Watts

9. Modern ECT differs from older and more extreme versions of the procedure in all of the following ways except
    a. the electrical charge used today is of lower voltage.
    b. the electrical charge used today is of shorter duration.
    c. today, electrodes are placed on both sides of the head, not just on one side, as was done in the past.
    d. today, a general anesthetic, a muscle relaxant and oxygen are administered as part of the procedure.

10. What kinds of mental disorders are treated with ECT today?
    a. severe mood disorders
    b. severe schizophrenia
    c. mild cases of schizophrenia
    d. agoraphobia and panic disorder

Answers to test your understanding

1. a. (15-1)
2. b. (15-1)
3. b. (15-1)
4. c. (15-2)
5. d. (15-2)
6. a. (15-3)
7. c. (15-3)
8. b. (15-4)
9. c. (15-4)
10. a. (15-4)

15-5	Why is the use of psychoactive drug therapy increasing in popularity?

14. In the 1950's, the introduction of medications called psychoactive or _____ (psychotropic / illegal) drugs gave rise to the scientific field of _____ (bio-psychiatry / psychopharmacology), which was devoted to the study of psychoactive drugs and their use in treating mental disorders. The prescription of psychotropic medication for mental disorders has been steadily _____ (decreasing / increasing). In 1975, _____ (only 27 / up to 90) percent of psychiatric

outpatients were given drugs. By 1988, that figure had _____ (dropped / grown) to 55 percent. Today, psychiatrists prescribe psychotropic medication for _____ (only 27 / up to 90) percent of their patients.

15. What are three reasons for the increasing popularity of drug therapies?

a.

b.

c.

15-6   How do psychoactive drugs work?

---

16. In your own words, briefly describe four ways that psychoactive drugs can modify the action of neurotransmitters in the brain.

a.

b.

c.

d.

17. Why are there side effects associated with most psychotropic drugs?

15-7	What medications are commonly used to treat mood disorders? How do they work?

18. Fill in the missing information about antidepressant medications.

DRUG CLASS	MODE OF ACTION	POSSIBLE SIDE EFFECTS
MAO Inhibitors		
Tricylics		
SSRIs		
Heterocyclic Antidepressants		

19. a.   What should be remembered when considering the use of antidepressants for

    1.   the elderly?

    2.   children and adolescents?

    b.   Can the long-term use of antidepressants result in physical addiction?

20. a.   What is the most commonly prescribed mood stabilizer used to treat bipolar disorder?

    b.   Describe two theories of its mode of action.

          1.

          2.

    c.   Is it effective?

    d.   Lithium is often used as a prophylactic drug. What does that mean?

| 15-8 | What medications are commonly used in the treatment of anxiety disorders? How do they work? |

21. Fill in the missing information about antianxiety agents.

DRUG CLASS	MODE OF ACTION	POSSIBLE SIDE EFFECTS
Benzodiazepines		
Nonbenzodiazepine Anxiolytics (Buspirone)		

22. In your own words, briefly describe the role of antidepressant medication in the treatment of anxiety.

> 15-9   What medications are commonly used in the treatment of schizophrenia? How do
> they work?

23. Fill in the missing information about antipsychotic agents.

DRUG CLASS	MODE OF ACTION	POSSIBLE SIDE EFFECTS
Typical Neuroleptics (Phenothiazines)		
Atypical Neuroleptics (Clozapine)		

> 15-10   What medications are commonly used in the treatment of attention-deficit/
> hyperactivity disorder? How do they work?

24. Briefly describe the mode of action of the following psychostimulants.

    a.   methylphenidate (Ritalin)

    b.   pemoline (Cylert)

25. What are the possible physical side effects of psychostimulant use?

26. In your own words, briefly describe some of the concerns of the long-term use of psychostimulants.

> 15-11   How do ethnicity and gender relate to psychoactive drugs?

27. In your own words, briefly discuss how ethnicity relates to the effects of the following medications.

    a.   tricyclic antidepressants

    b.   benzodiazepines

    c.   neuroleptics

28. In your own words, briefly discuss the possible impact of gender on the effects of psychotropic drugs.

Test your understanding

1. The use of psychotropic drugs in the treatment of mental disorders has
   a. increased dramatically between 1950 and 1990, but has decreased in the last few years.
   b. decreased dramatically between 1950 and 1990, but has increased in the last few years.
   c. decreased steadily for the last 50 years.
   d. increased steadily for the last 50 years.

2. An agonist is
   a. a person in great pain.
   b. a psychoactive drug which enhances neural activity because it is chemically similar enough to a natural neurotransmitter to mimic its effects.
   c. a psychoactive drug which reduces neuronal activity by attaching to and blocking the natural neurotransmitter's receptor site.
   d. a psychoactive drug which enhances neuronal activity by blocking the reuptake of various neurotransmitters.

3. An antagonist is
   a. a anaesthetic used in ECT.
   b. a psychoactive drug which enhances neural activity because it is chemically similar enough to a natural neurotransmitter to mimic its effects.
   c. a psychoactive drug which reduces neuronal activity by attaching to and blocking the natural neurotransmitter's receptor site.
   d. a psychoactive drug which enhances neuronal activity by blocking the reuptake of various neurotransmitters.

4. Which of the following is not a class of antidepressant medication?
   a. MAO inhibitors
   b. tricyclics
   c. selective serotonin reuptake inhibitors (SSRIs)
   d. benzodiazepines

5. Lithium carbonate is
    a. a MAO inhibitor.
    b. the most commonly prescribed mood stabilizer used to treat bipolar disorder.
    c. the most commonly prescribed mood stabilizer used to treat major depression and dysthymic disorder.
    d. a commonly used drug to treat chronic anxiety and in some cases, panic attacks.

6. Benzodiazepines
    a. reduce anxiety by increasing the effects of GABA, an inhibitory neurotransmitter.
    b. reduce anxiety by decreasing the effects of dopamine.
    c. reduce anxiety by blocking the reuptake of serotonin.
    d. reduce anxiety by destroying monoamine oxidase.

7. Typical neuroleptics (phenothiazines)
    a. are dopamine agonists.
    b. are dopamine antagonists.
    c. are serotonin reuptake inhibitors.
    d. do not cause serious side effects.

8. Which of the following are not possible negative side effects of typical neuroleptics?
    a. acute dystonia
    b. tardive dyskinesia
    c. agranulocytosis
    d. neuroleptic malignant syndrome

9. Which drug, sometimes used in the treatment of attention-deficit/hyperactivity disorder works by mimicking the neurotransmitter dopamine?
    a. pemoline (Cylert)
    b. fluoxetine (Prozac)
    c. nefazodone (Serzone)
    d. bupropion (Wellbutrin)

10. Which ethnic and gender groups are generally most sensitive to psychotropic drugs?
    a. men and European Caucasians
    b. women and European Caucasians
    c. men and African Americans
    d. women and Asians

Answers to test your understanding

1. d.   (15-5)
2. b.   (15-6)
3. c.   (15-6)
4. d.   (15-7)
5. b.   (15-7)
6. a.   (15-8)
7. b.   (15-9)
8. c.   (15-9)
9. a.   (15-10)
10. d.   (15-11)

When you have finished . . .

Explore the Web to find more information

The **American Psychological Association** offers an excellent article on electroconvulsive therapy (ECT). You can access it at (**http://www.psych.org/public_info/ECT~1.HTM**).

Another good link for more information on electroconvulsive therapy is offered at **ECT On-line**. (**http://www.priory.co.uk/journals/psych/ectol.htm**) When you get to their site, click on, Patient Information Leaflet (Royal College of Psychiatrists). You will also find a link to other ECT links, some opposing the use of ECT.

A very informative document which is part of the Decade of the Brain Series, is distributed by **The National Institutes of Mental Health**. It is titled, "Medications - Mental Health/Mental Illness." Access it at (**gopher://gopher.nimh.nih.gov:70/00/documents/nimh/other/Medicate**).

Internet Mental Health has a very complete database for psychotherapeutic drug information. You will find information on each medication in the database including:
    pharmacology
    indications
    contraindications
    warnings
    precautions
    adverse effects
    overdose
    dosage
    supplied
    research
Access this database at (**http://www.mentalhealth.com/fr30.html**).

"What Is Neuroleptic Malignant Syndrome?" is an article taken from The Harvard Medical School Mental Health Letter, October, 1987. It is provided by **Internet Mental Health** and can be accessed by going to (**http://www.mentalhealth.com/mag1/p5h-nms1.html**).

CHAPTER 16
Psychotherapy

Before you read . . .

Survey the chapter

Chapter 16 focuses on some of the major types of psychotherapy. As you read this chapter, you will find more than just a listing of different therapeutic techniques. Important questions concerning the effectiveness of psychotherapy are discussed. Does psychotherapy work? If so, why does it sometimes help people? Is successful treatment determined most by the skill, knowledge and experience of the therapist, the specific method used or perhaps the relationship between the clinician and client? How do we know which techniques are more effective than others? Can psychotherapy be studied in a laboratory? Can it be studied at all?

As you read . . .

Ask questions

16-1   What kinds of people are most likely to seek out and benefit from psychotherapy?

16-2   What are the most important components of successful psychotherapy?

16-3   What are the major theoretical models used in psychotherapy? Which ones are the most popular?

16-4   What are the goals and techniques of traditional Freudian psychoanalysis?

16-5   What are some of the therapeutic variations of traditional psychoanalysis?

16-6   What are the goals and techniques of interpersonal therapies?

16-7   What are the goals and techniques of phenomenological/experiential (P/E) therapies?

16-8   What are the goals and techniques of behavioral therapies?

16-9   What are the goals and techniques of cognitive therapies?

16-10   What methods are used to evaluate the effectiveness of psychotherapy?

16-11   Why is it that psychotherapy researchers have such a problem with validity when conducting their studies?

16-12   How do researchers study the effects of psychotherapy and what have they found?

After you read . . .

Review and explore the chapter

> 16-1   What kinds of people are most likely to seek out and benefit from psychotherapy?

1.   Psychotherapists, whether they be psychiatrists, psychologists, clinical social workers, pastoral counselors, psychiatric nurses or other counselors, are expected to have three attributes. What are they?

a. *Special training + experience treating people*

b. *Ability to show empathy for the client*

c. *Capacity for warmly supporting clients.*

2.   Are age and gender related to the effectiveness of psychotherapy?   *No*

3.   Is socioeconomic status related to the effectiveness of psychotherapy? If so, how?

Yes. People from lower socioeconomic groups tend to seek psychotherapy less often + terminate therapy earlier than persons in higher socioeconomic statuses.

4. Why is it important that therapists conduct psychotherapy in a culturally sensitive manner?

Clients from different cultural backgrounds have different values + beliefs, which can have a dramatic impact on their ability to participate + succeed in therapy.

5. a. Which one of the following ethnic groups, African Americans, Asian Americans, European Americans or Hispanic Americans, tends to receive mental health services most frequently?

   b. Which two of the above groups tend to receive mental health services least frequently?

   Hispanic Americans

   Asian Americans

6. Below is a list of a few of the types of problems most commonly treated in psychotherapy. Rank them from 1-5 in order of frequency.

   a. __5__ mental retardation
   b. __3__ physical complaints
   c. __4__ psychotic conditions
   d. __1__ anxiety and depression
   e. __2__ interpersonal and marital problems

   1. anxiety / depression
   2. interpersonal / marital problems
   3. physical complaints
   4. psychotic conditions
   5. mental retardation

16-2	What are the most important components of successful psychotherapy?

7. a. What does research tell us about the differences in effectiveness between professionally trained therapists and nonprofessional counselors?

   Clients treated by nonprofessional counselors do about as well as persons treated by professional therapists.

   b. What does research tell us about the differences in effectiveness between experienced and novice therapists?

   Novice therapists do about as well as experienced therapists.

8. a. In your own words, briefly discuss the single most critical component of successful psychotherapy.

   most crucial component: relationship between client + therapist.

b.   What can therapists do to help foster the development of a positive therapeutic bond?

They can develop an initial therapeutic contract, seek to maintain conditions which will facilitate the continued growth of the therapeutic relationship + act in a professional manner.

16-3   What are the major theoretical models used in psychotherapy? Which ones are the most popular?

---

9.   What are the five major theoretical models which guide most psychotherapeutic techniques?

a. *psychoanalytic / psychodynamic*

b. *phenomenological / experiental*

c. *interpersonal*

d. *behavioral*

e. *cognitive - behavioral*

10. a.   Most therapists describe themselves as eclectic or integrationist. What does this mean?

They combine the assumptions + procedures from 2 or more theoretical points of view.

b.   What are the most popular theoretical components among eclectic therapists?

In descending order:
1. psychodynamic
2. cognitive
3. behavioral
4. phenomenological / experimental

16-4   What are the goals and techniques of traditional Freudian psychoanalysis?

11. The primary goal of Freudian psychoanalysis is to help clients understand the *unconscious* (conscious / unconscious) reasons why they act in maladaptive ways. The problem(s) would disappear when understanding and acceptance were achieved. The therapy, which can take *years* (weeks / months / years), involves two types of self-exploration. The first is *insight* (insight / repression) or recognition of the long-hidden problems, followed by *emotionally* (intellectual / emotionally *working through*) understanding of (emotionally working through) this new found awareness in order to understand how the repressed problems are still affecting the client's life.

12. Match the following concepts taken from the major techniques used in psychoanalysis.

1. *a* free association
2. *d* latent dream content
3. *f* manifest dream content
4. *h* interpretation of everyday behavior
5. *b* resistance
6. *e* transference
7. *g* transference neurosis
8. *c* countertransference

free association a. requires that the client say everything that comes to mind without censoring it

resistance b. client tries to avoid coming to grips with previously unconscious, conflict-filled and threatening material

counter-transference c. the therapist's own unconscious feelings towards the client which may distort the analytic process

latent dream content d. the obvious features of a dream, not as important in analysis as other dream content

transference e. client begins to unconsciously attach characteristics of significant people from the past to the therapist and begins to reenact reactions, conflicts and impulses associated with those important figures

manifest dream content f. the unconsciousness ideas and impulses symbolized in a dream

transference neurosis g. type of transference which is a miniaturized version of the patient's problems

interpretation of everyday behavior h. used because unconscious conflicts and defenses may be reflected in slips-of-the-tongue, jokes or seemingly simple forgetfulness

| 16-5 | What are some of the therapeutic variations of traditional psychoanalysis? |

13. Fill in the missing information in the table below.

VARIATIONS OF PSYCHOANALYSIS	
THERAPY	MAJOR GOALS / TECHNIQUES
Psychoanalytically Oriented Psychotherapy	
Ego Analysis	
Adler's Individual Psychology	
Object Relations and Self Therapy	

| 16-6 | What are the goals and techniques of interpersonal therapies? |

14. In your own words, briefly describe Harry Stack Sullivan's interpersonal therapy.

15. In your own words briefly describe Weissman and Klerman's form of interpersonal therapy.

Test your understanding

1. Which of the following is not an attribute expected of all psychotherapists, whether they be psychiatrists, psychologists, clinical social workers, pastoral counselors or psychiatric nurses?
    a. special training and experience treating people
    b. the ability to show empathy for the client
    c. the capacity for warmly supporting clients.
    d. a Ph.D. degree

2. Which of the following client attributes is most related to the effectiveness of therapy?
    a. age
    b. gender
    c. socioeconomic status
    d. intelligence

3. The most commonly treated problems in psychotherapy are
    a. anxiety and depression.
    b. physical complaints.
    c. psychotic conditions.
    d. interpersonal and marital problems.

4. Which of the following statements about the effectiveness of psychotherapy is true?
    a. Professionally trained psychotherapists are much more effective than are nonprofessional counselors.
    b. Experienced psychotherapists are much more effective than novice therapists.
    c. The amount of professional training and experience of the therapist does not strongly relate to the effectiveness of therapy.
    d. Whether the clinician is professionally trained and experienced or not, psychotherapy is rarely effective.

5. What is the single most critical component of successful psychotherapy?
    a. the training of the therapist
    b. the client-therapist relationship
    c. the match between therapeutic method and disorder
    d. the willingness of the client to change

6. A therapist describes her techniques as eclectic. This means that
    a. the therapy will be expensive.
    b. she is a classically-trained psychoanalyst.
    c. she uses a combination of assumptions and procedures taken from different theoretical approaches.
    d. the client will be treated with respect, positive regard and empathy.

7. The most popular theoretical components among eclectic therapists are
    a. psychodynamic, cognitive, behavioral and phenomenological/experiential.
    b. behavioral, interpersonal and hypnotherapy.
    c. Gestalt, ego analysis and object relations self therapy.
    d. biofeedback, modeling and systematic desensitization therapy.

8. In traditional psychoanalytic therapy, the unconscious ideas and impulses symbolized in a dream are called
    a. the manifest content of the dream.
    b. the latent content of the dream.
    c. symbolized dream content.
    d. neurotic dream content.

9. Which technique in traditional psychoanalysis requires the client to say everything that comes to mind without censoring it?
    a. transference
    b. countertransference

c. interpretation of everyday behavior

d. free association

10. The process in psychoanalytic therapy where the client begins to unconsciously attach characteristics of significant people from the past to the therapist and begins to reenact reactions, conflicts and impulses associated with those important figures is

a. transference.

b. countertransference.

c. transference neurosis.

d. free association.

11. The usual psychoanalytically oriented psychotherapy of today differs from Freud's original version in that

a. it is more likely to use biological techniques such as biofeedback.

b. it is less likely to make use of biological techniques such as biofeedback.

c. it is more formal, less flexible and lasts longer.

d. it is less formal, more flexible, lasts less time and is more conversational in style.

12. Object relations and self therapy emphasizes

a. conscious over unconscious needs.

b. the ego's role in the inability to develop positive adaptive behavior.

c. the long-term effects of the infant and caregiver's relationship.

d. the use of dream analysis and direct advice to help the client combat mistaken beliefs about the self and build a new lifestyle.

13. Adler's individual psychology emphasizes

a. conscious over unconscious needs.

b. the ego's role in the inability to develop positive adaptive behavior.

c. the long-term effects of the infant and caregiver's relationship.

d. the use of dream analysis and direct advice to help the client combat

mistaken beliefs about the self and build a new lifestyle.

14. The goal of Sullivan's interpersonal therapy is to

a. enhance the client's ability to be open, honest, flexible and positive with others.

b. uncover repressed feelings and impulses which were brought about by problematic relationships with others.

c. help clients be less dependent on others.

d. help clients be more dependent on others.

15. Which of the following is not a potentially problematic interpersonal situation which can relate to depression according to Weissman and Klerman's version of interpersonal therapy?

a. prolonged grieving over the loss of a loved one

b. nonconflicting demands of social roles

c. difficult transitions

d. lack of social skills

Answers to test your understanding

1.	d.	(16-1)
2.	c.	(16-1)
3.	a.	(16-1)
4.	c.	(16-2)
5.	b.	(16-2)
6.	c.	(16-3)
7.	a.	(16-3)
8.	b.	(16-4)
9.	d.	(16-4)
10.	a.	(16-4)
11.	d.	(16-5)
12.	c.	(16-5)
13.	d.	(16-5)
14.	a.	(16-6)
15.	d.	(16-6)

16-7   What are the goals and techniques of phenomenological/experiential (P/E) therapies?

---

16. Each of the following statements about the basic assumptions of phenomenological/experiential approach is not true. Rewrite each statement to make it correct.

a.   Phenomenologists believe that the client must learn to see and understand the world through the eyes of the therapist.

b.   P/E therapists have a negative view of human beings and believe that people are driven by instinct. Therefore, there is no such thing as free will.

c.   P/E therapists believe that the most important factor in successful therapy is the skill of the therapist in making the client understand that certain behaviors will not be tolerated.

d.   It is important, P/E therapists believe, that patients understand that the therapist is in charge, if treatment is to be successful.

e.   P/E therapy is based on the changing of behavior. The experience and exploration of painful or confusing emotions only gets in the way.

17. Describe the empty chair technique.

18. a.   In client-centered therapy, how do "conditions of worth" retard personal growth?

b.   What type of therapeutic relationship do client-centered therapists believe is necessary to avoid imposing conditions of worth on the client?

c.   What three interrelated attitudes, known as facilitative conditions, are communicated to the client in order to allow personal growth to resume?

1.

2.

3.

19. In your own words, briefly discuss Gestalt therapy.

16-8   What are the goals and techniques of behavioral therapies?

---

20. How has behavior therapy changed in the last twenty years?

21. In the table below, briefly describe in your own words, each of the following behaviorally based therapies.

BEHAVIORALLY-BASED THERAPY		DESCRIPTION OF MAJOR FOCUS / ELEMENTS
Systematic Desensitization		
Exposure Treatments		
Assertiveness Training		
Modeling	Modeling	
	Coping Modeling	
Contingency Management		
Contingency Contracting	Contingency Contracting	
	Token Economy	
Biofeedback		
Aversion Therapy		

16-9   What are the goals and techniques of cognitive therapies?

22. What is the major difference between the focus of cognitive therapy (also called cognitive-behavioral therapy) and the traditional behavioral therapies like those above?

23. In your own words, briefly describe the focus and main elements of Beck's cognitive therapy.

24. In your own words, briefly describe the focus and main elements of Ellis's rational emotive therapy (RET).

16-10   What methods are used to evaluate the effectiveness of psychotherapy?

25. In the most basic type of psychotherapy outcome experiment, clients displaying the same type of disorder are _____ (randomly / carefully) assigned to either a no-treatment or _____ (experimental / control) group and a treatment or _____ (experimental / control) group. After assignment is made, the _____ (independent / dependent) variable, such as anxiety level or depression, is measured and compared for the two groups. In more elaborate experiments, called _____ (factorial designs / confounded experiments), more than one variable can be manipulated and studied.

26. a.   Why have placebo groups been commonly used as a control in psychotherapy research?

    b.   What are three problems associated with the use of placebo groups in research?

        1.

        2.

        3.

27. Another scientific approach to evaluating the effects of psychotherapy is the within-subject experiment, which measures changes that occur in _____ (the same client / different clients) at _____ (the same time / different times). In the simplest within-subject design, a _____

(value free / baseline) measurement of specific behaviors is made followed by an _____ (intervention / independent variable retraction) phase in which treatment is given. In some cases, for added experimental control, a no-treatment baseline condition is alternated with treatment. This is called an _____ (ABAB / double exposure) design.

28. a.   What is a single subject or N=1 study?

     b.   List four reason why N=1 research is increasing in popularity.

           1.

           2.

           3.

           4.

16-11	Why is it that psychotherapy researchers have such a problem with validity when conducting their studies?

29. Match the following.

     1.   ____ internal validity
     2.   ____ external validity
     3.   ____ statistical validity

           a.   refers to whether there were enough subjects in the experiment to allow statistical analysis to detect any significant differences between group differences

           b.   the degree to which an experiment's results can be generalized to a larger population

    c.   the degree to which an experimenter can be confident that the results are due to the independent variable and not some other factor or factors

30.   What are four options that researchers have which can help them deal with threats to validity in their experiments?

    a.

    b.

    c.

    d.

31.   Is it easy for researchers to construct research designs which have a high degree of internal, external and statistical validity simultaneously?

16-12   How do researchers study the effects of psychotherapy and what have they found?

32.   What is meta-analysis and what role has it played in the controversy surrounding the value of psychotherapy?

33.   What five conclusions about the effectiveness of psychotherapy can be drawn from meta-analysis?

    a.

b.

c.

d.

e.

Test your understanding

1. Which of the following statements about phenomenological/experiential therapy is true?
    a. Phenomenologists believe that the client must learn to see and understand the world through the eyes of the therapist.
    b. P/E therapists have a negative view of human beings and believe that people are driven by instinct.
    c. P/E therapists believe it is important, if treatment is to be successful, that patients understand that the therapist is in charge.
    d. P/E therapy emphasizes the experience and exploration of painful or confusing emotions as important to the therapeutic process.

2. Conditions of worth are
    a. healthy self-images which are the goal of client-centered therapy.
    b. judgements imposed by others which distort an individual's feelings and actions and hamper personal growth and well being.
    c. contracts, drawn up between therapist and client, which spell out needed changes in behavior and thinking.
    d. a list of ten separate goal behaviors used by client-centered therapists.

3. Which of the following is not an important aspect of the therapist's relationship with the client in client-centered therapy?
    a. unconditional positive regard of the client by the therapist
    b. warm, but firm correction of the client's improper behaviors by the therapist
    c. empathetic understanding on the part of the therapist
    d. the therapist's actions and feelings must be genuine and congruent

4. How has behavior therapy changed in the last twenty years?
    a. It has broadened its focus to reflect the latest research in perception, cognition and biological bases of behavior.
    b. It has broadened its focus to reflect the latest developments in our understanding of the subconscious.
    c. Twenty years ago behavioral therapy was quite popular. Today, it is rarely used.
    d. Twenty years ago, behavioral therapy was rarely used. Today, it is quite popular.

5. Which behaviorally-based method, commonly used to treat phobias and other anxiety problems, uses relaxation coupled with gradual exposure to a hierarchy of anxiety-arousing stimuli?
    a. exposure treatments
    b. modeling
    c. aversive therapy
    d. systematic desensitization

6. Which controversial behaviorally-based technique uses the presentation of painful or unpleasant stimuli in hopes of decreasing unwanted behaviors?
    a. exposure treatments
    b. modeling
    c. aversive therapy
    d. systematic desensitization

7. Which behaviorally-based method relies on the client observing others engaging successfully in feared behaviors?
    a. exposure treatments
    b. modeling
    c. aversive therapy
    d. systematic desensitization

8. What is the major difference between the focus of cognitive (cognitive-behavioral) therapy and traditional behavioristic therapy?
    a. Cognitive therapy focuses on the maladaptive thoughts and beliefs which traditional behavioristic therapy tends to ignore.
    b. Traditional behavioristic therapy focuses on the maladaptive thoughts and beliefs which cognitive therapy tends to ignore.
    c. Dream analysis is an important part of cognitive therapy, but not of behavioristic therapy.
    d. Overt behavior, which is the focus of behavior therapy, is of no importance to a cognitive therapist.

9. According to Ellis' rational emotive therapy, upsetting emotions and other problems are often the result of
    a. the long-term effects of poor parenting.
    b. the long-term effects of chronic stress.
    c. irrational, extreme and self-defeating beliefs.
    d. problematic interpersonal relationships brought on by a lack of social skills.

10. In a psychotherapy outcome experiment, assignment to either a treatment or no-treatment group is
    a. usually dependent on the age of the client subject.
    b. usually dependent on the gender of the client subject.
    c. usually dependent on the ethnicity of the client subject.
    d. random.

11. Within-subject experiments
    a. measure changes that occur in placebo subjects and compare the results to the experimental treatment group.
    b. measure changes in different subjects at the same time.
    c. measure changes in the same subject at different times.
    d. measure changes in the same subject only once.

12. Single-subject or N=1 studies
    a. were outlawed by the federal
        government in 1959.
    b. use only one subject for research.
    c. use one single variable per subject for
        research.
    d. use one subject for both experimental
        and control purposes.

13. External validity
    a. refers to whether there were enough
        subjects in the experiment to allow
        statistical analysis to detect any
        significant differences between group
        differences.
    b. refers to the degree to which an
        experiment's results can be generalized
        to a larger population.
    c. refers to the degree to which an
        experimenter can be confident that the
        results are due to the independent
        variable and not some other factor.
    d. refers to the degree to which the results
        for the experimental group can be
        compared to the control or placebo
        group.

14. Is it easy to construct research designs
    which have a high degree of internal,
    external and statistical validity
    simultaneously?
    a. Yes, because if validity is high in one
        type, the others will be high also.
    b. Yes, because psychotherapeutic
        research is relatively easy to design,
        compared to other types of research.
    c. No, because it is almost impossible to
        design therapy outcome research which
        will be high in any of the three types of
        validity.
    d. No, because outcome research which is
        designed to maximize one form of
        validity, often precludes high degrees
        of other types of experimental validity.

15. An important finding of meta-analysis is
    that
    a. psychotherapy doesn't work for most
        people.
    b. the average person receiving
        psychotherapy is better off than 80
        percent of the persons who did not
        receive therapy.
    c. five years after the end of therapy most
        persons have deteriorated back to their
        formal levels of disorder.
    d. the higher the level of experience and
        training of the therapist, the higher the
        success rates of the therapy.

Answers to test your understanding

1. d. (16-7)
2. b. (16-7)
3. b. (16-7)
4. a. (16-8)
5. d. (16-8)
6. c. (16-8)
7. b. (16-8)
8. a. (16-9)
9. c. (16-9)
10. d. (16-10)
11. c. (16-10)
12. b. (16-10)
13. b. (16-11)
14. d. (16-11)
15. b. (16-11)

When you have finished . . .

Explore the Web to find more information

A good general discussion of therapy can be found in a publication designed for the general public by **The American Psychological Association**. The article, **"Finding Help: How to Choose a Psychologist,"** can be accessed at (**http://www.apa.org/pubinfo/howto.html**).

The American Psychoanalytic Association home page is located at (**http://198.69.121.38/**). Follow the link, About Psychoanalysis for general information.

Internet Mental Health offers the following articles:

*   "Behavior Therapy," The Harvard Mental Health Letter, December, 1990 (Part I), January, 1991 (Part II). (**http://www.mentalhealth.com/mag1/p5h-beh1.html**)

*   "Cognitive Therapy," The Harvard Medical School Mental Health Letter, August (Part I), September, 1989 (Part II). (**http://www.mentalhealth.com/mag1/p5h-cog1.html**)

The home page of **The Albert Ellis Institute**, (formerly known as the **Institute for Rational-Emotive Therapy**) is located at (**http://www.IRET.org/**). Click on, Questions and Answers about Rational Emotive Behavior Therapy or you can even submit a question directly to Dr. Ellis. One question is answered each month.

In this chapter, you read about how essential it is that therapists conduct psychotherapy in a culturally sensitive manner. At (**http://www.apa.org/pi/guide.html**) you will find the **American Psychological Association's**, "Guidelines for Providers of Psychological Services to Ethnic, Linguistic and Culturally Diverse Populations."

You can read more about the effectiveness of psychotherapy and the Consumer Reports Study in the **Internet Mental Health** Article, "Long-Term Psychotherapy Is Highly Effective: The Consumer Reports Study," by Martin E. P. Seligman, The Harvard Mental Health Letter, July, 1996. The URL is (**http://www.mentalhealth.com/mag1/p5h-rx02.html**).

CHAPTER 17
Alternatives to Individual Psychotherapy

Before you read . . .

Survey the chapter

Chapter 17 begins with the case of Juan, a man who immigrated to the United States at age thirteen. Juan's life was not an easy one; subjected to a variety of cultural and socioeconomic stressors and dealing with the onset of schizophrenia, Juan deteriorated over the next 20 years. During that time Juan repeatedly came into contact with traditional metal health services, but they were of no substantial help. Could something have been done differently?

This chapter looks at possible alternatives to individual psychotherapy. These approaches focus on how other people contribute to or are affected by disturbed behavior and efforts to provide self-help and rehabilitation services. These alternative approaches often differ from traditional psychotherapy in two important ways. First, they attempt to prevent or at least lessen the effects of mental illness by developing programs which are designed to change maladaptive environments. Secondly, they attempt to empower those individuals whose life circumstances have placed them at a greater risk for developing mental disorders.

As you read . . .

Ask questions

17-1   If individual psychotherapy is effective for most clients, why do we need alternative psychological interventions?

17-2   What is group therapy?

17-3   Is group therapy an effective form of treatment?

17-4   Are there alternative forms of therapy designed to help couples?

17-5   Is marital/couples therapy an effective form of treatment?

17-6   What are the goals and techniques of family therapy?

17-7   Is family therapy an effective form of treatment?

17-8   What are self-help groups?

17-9   Can membership in self-help groups be therapeutic?

17-10   What is psychosocial rehabilitation?

17-11   Can psychosocial rehabilitation effectively help severely mentally ill patients?

17-12   What is community psychology?

17-13   In what ways does community psychology attempt to promote the prevention of mental health problems?

17-14   If they are going to work, how must prevention programs be designed?

After you read . . .

Review and explore the chapter

> 17-1   If individual psychotherapy is effective for most clients, why do we need alternative psychological interventions?

1.   Match the following.

1   _d_ group therapy
2   _c_ marital or couples therapy
3.   _a_ family therapy
4.   _e_ psychosocial rehabilitation programs
5.   _b_ primary prevention programs

   a.   focuses on how forces within the family affect the functioning of each of its members

   b.   attempts to modify social, economic and environmental factors that lead to dysfunction, while also strengthening those positive qualities which can help protect individuals from developing mental disorders

   c.   addresses problems involved in the intimate interactions among couples

   d.   seeks changes in the way individuals tend to interact in a wide range of interpersonal relationships

e. helps people with mental disorders cope with the occupational, economic, family and environmental effects of his or her disorder

2. What is meant when it is said that the alternatives to individual therapy are a more social therapy than psychotherapy?

3. Proponents of alternative therapies often point out that access to individual psychotherapy may be limited to some people. Discuss three factors which may account for limited access.

   a. *Too expensive*

   b. *reluctant because of perceived stigma*

   c. *not enough health care professionals available to give help to those who need it.*

4. Proponents of alternative forms of therapy often point out that individual psychotherapy assumes that something inside the client needs to change. Why do they see this as a problem?

5. Proponents of a prevention over treatment approach in dealing with mental disorder often argue that individual psychotherapy places too much emphasis on psychopathology. Why do they see this as a problem and where do they believe the emphasis should lie?

17-2   What is group therapy?

6. a. Define group therapy in your own words.

b.   What event had the effect of increasing the use and popularity of group therapy?

c.   Which of the major theoretical approaches to individual therapy are also commonly offered in a group format?

d.   Do nonprofessional and self-help groups use group therapy?

7.   Some therapy groups employ the same specific techniques used in individual forms of therapy. If the methods are the same, what does the group format add to the therapeutic experience?

8.   Other kinds of group therapy are based on the premise that the interactions and experiences that clients have within the group itself are the most important elements in their therapeutic success. Briefly discuss eight different therapeutic factors which occur in an ideal group setting.

a.

b.

c.

d.

e.

f.

g.

h.

9. Therapy groups usually consist of _____ (6 to 12 / 20 to 30) members. Some groups are _____ (homogeneous / heterogeneous), consisting of members who are similar in age, gender or type of problem. Some groups are _____ (homogeneous / heterogeneous), consisting of members who are dissimilar. Group sessions usually last about _____ (half / twice) as long as individual psychotherapy sessions, with the group meeting for as little as a few sessions to, in some cases, years. Group therapy is becoming _____ (increasingly / decreasingly) popular because it is _____ (less / more) expensive than its individual therapy counterpart.

10. a.   Does the therapy group leader's experience, training, leadership style or theoretical background typically affect the outcome of group treatments?

    b.   What are the characteristics of an effective group leader?

17-3	Is group therapy an effective form of treatment?

11. a.   Can group therapy be an effective form of treatment?

    b.   What elements increase the effectiveness of therapy groups?

c.   Is individual psychotherapy more effective than group therapy?

17-4   Are there alternative forms of therapy designed to help couples?

12. a.   Define marital therapy (also known as couples therapy) in your own words.

psychological treatment of problems in marriage + other intimate relationships.

b.   According to your text, who is the true client in couples therapy?

the relationship)

c.   What is conjoint therapy?

when both members of a relationship see the same therapist in the same sessions)

13.   In your own words, briefly discuss the goals and techniques used in the following types of marital therapy.

a.   behaviorally-based therapies, such as behavioral exchange contracts

rewarding wanted target behaviors which they believe will aid the relationship; not reinforcing unwanted problematic actions

b.   cognitive-behavioral oriented therapies

focus on ways a couple thinks about their relationship & attempts to modify the attributions the couple makes about each other.

c.   emotionally-focused couples therapy

tries to help partners feel more comfortable expressing & accepting each other's emotional needs

d.   insight-oriented couples therapy

focuses on unconscious conflicts in the relationship)

e.   communications training *used by almost all therapists*

teaches couple to inter more openly & honestly in order to be able to solve problems together.

17-5	Is marital/couples therapy an effective form of treatment?

14. Are the following statements about the effects of marital therapy true or false? If the statement is incorrect, change it to make it true.

   a. Compared with no-treatment control groups, almost all forms of marital therapy can produce significant improvement in a couple's happiness and adjustment.

   T

   b. Even when improvements are made, as many as ~~90~~ *50* percent of treated relationships remain distressed.

   F

   c. Approximately 30-40 percent of couples treated with behavioral marital techniques, relapse into marital discord or divorce.

   T

   d. Unlike marital therapy, marital enrichment programs have *not* ~~consistently been~~ shown to produce lasting changes in long-term relationships.

   F

   e. No specific type of marital therapy is better than any other in terms of effectiveness and success.

   T

17-6	What are the goals and techniques of family therapy?

15. Define family therapy in your own words.

   aimed at changing family interaction to correct family disturbances

16. What are the three principles of systems theory? How does each relate to family interaction?

   a. *circular cause*

b. *ecology — look at the whole picture*

c. *Subjectivity — ea person has his own perception of events*

17. Who is the identified client in family therapy?

The one member of the most easily identified problems

18. Why is communication among family members a common focal point in family therapy?

✓ is often via threats & other coercive messages

19. In your own words, briefly describe each of the following techniques commonly used in family therapy.

   a.   behaviorally-based family therapies

   b.   strategic or structural family therapy

   c.   paradoxical directives

17-7	Is family therapy an effective form of treatment?

20. a.   Is family therapy an effective treatment for some disorders and family problems?

Yes

   b.   Which two types of family therapy seem to be more effective than others?

Test your understanding

1. The alternative to individual psychotherapy which attempts to (1) modify social, economic and environmental factors that lead to dysfunction and (2) strengthen positive qualities which can help protect individuals from developing mental disorders is
    a. group therapy.
    b. marital or couples therapy.
    c. psychosocial rehabilitation programs.
    d. primary prevention programs.

2. The alternative to individual psychotherapy which seeks changes in the way individuals tend to interact in a wide range of interpersonal relationships is
    a. group therapy.
    b. marital or couples therapy.
    c. psychosocial rehabilitation programs.
    d. primary prevention programs.

3. The alternative to individual psychotherapy which helps people with mental disorders cope with the occupational, economic, family and environmental effects of his or her disorder is
    a. group therapy.
    b. marital or couples therapy.
    c. psychosocial rehabilitation programs.
    d. primary prevention programs.

4. Proponents of alternative therapies often point out that access to individual psychotherapy may be limited for some persons. Which of the following is not one of their arguments?
    a. Individual psychotherapy is often expensive and many people can't afford it.
    b. Many people are reluctant to seek psychotherapy because of cultural values or perceived stigma.
    c. Individual psychotherapy is unavailable in most rural areas of the United States.
    d. There are not enough health care professionals available to provide individual psychotherapy to all who need it.

5. Which of the following statements about group therapy is not true?
    a. The use of group therapy is increasing in popularity.
    b. Every major theoretical approach is offered in a group format.
    c. A major event which helped increase the popularity of group therapy was World War II.
    d. The group format is rarely used by nonprofessional or self-help groups because it is too complex.

6. All of the following therapeutic factors are part of the group therapy experience except
    a. the sharing of new information and insights with other members of the group.
    b. the fact that group feedback is powerful, especially if there is a variety of opinions from the members.
    c. the fact that group members learn that they are not the only ones who have problems in general or their kind of problem in particular.
    d. the fact that group members experience helping others.

7. Which of the following is the most important factor in the effectiveness of group leaders?
    a. the leader's understanding and knowledge of different therapeutic techniques
    b. the leader's understanding and knowledge and the chosen therapeutic technique
    c. the leader's experience with diverse

groups and group members

d. the leader's ability to accurately monitor the therapy process, communicate clearly with clients and convey warm support for clients

8. Can group therapy be an effective form of therapy?
   a. Yes, especially when the group members clearly understand how the group is run and what is expected of them.
   b. Yes, as long as the group has less than eight members.
   c. Yes, especially if the group leader has a Ph.D. degree and specialized therapeutic training.
   d. No, although group therapy can help a few people, it is never as effective as individual psychotherapy.

9. Who is the true client in marital (couples) therapy?
   a. the most dysfunctional member of the couple
   b. the identified client
   c. the relationship
   d. the person who most cares about the maintenance of the partnership

10. Which of the following is employed by almost all couples therapists?
    a. a behaviorally oriented couples contract
    b. communications training
    c. emotionally-focused couples therapy
    d. insight-oriented couples therapy

11. Which of the following statements about marital/couples therapy is true?
    a. Compared with no-treatment control groups, almost all forms of marital therapy can produce significant improvement in a couple's happiness and adjustment.
    b. Even when improvements are made, as many as 90 percent of treated

relationships remain distressed.

   c. It is rare for couples who have been successfully treated with behavioral marital techniques to relapse into marital discord or divorce.
   d. Unlike marital therapy, marital enrichment programs have consistently been shown to produce lasting changes in long-term relationships.

12. Which of the following is not an important aspect of systems theory?
    a. circular causality
    b. ecology
    c. subjectivity
    d. the principle of individual dominance

13. In family therapy, who is the identified client?
    a. the person of the family that is the cause of all of the family members' problems
    b. the one family member with the most easily identifiable problem
    c. the family member who first approaches a mental health professional and asks for help in dealing with another member's problem
    d. the relationship

14. Why is communication among family members a common focal point in family therapy?
    a. Most families don't talk, they just watch TV or ignore each other in other ways.
    b. Family members need good communication skills in order to convince the identified client that he or she needs help.
    c. In many disturbed families, the main communication methods involve threats and other coercive messages.
    d. Historically, most family therapists have had an interactionist perspective.

15. Which two types of family therapy seem to be more effective than others?
    a. psychodynamic and Gestalt based therapies
    b. interactionist and emotionally-focused therapy
    c. cognitive and cognitive-behavioral family therapies
    d. behavioral and structural family therapies

Answers to test your understanding

1.	d.	(17-1)
2.	a.	(17-1)
3.	c.	(17-1)
4.	c.	(17-1)
5.	d.	(17-2)
6.	b.	(17-2)
7.	d.	(17-2)
8.	a.	(17-3)
9.	c.	(17-4)
10.	b.	(17-4)
11.	a.	(17-5)
12.	d.	(17-6)
13.	b.	(17-6)
14.	c.	(17-6)
15.	d.	(17-7)

17-8   What are self-help groups?

---

21. Define self-help groups in your own words.

22. What four features are commonly shared by different self-help groups (SHGs)?

    a.

    b.

    c.

    d.

23. Match the following types of self-help groups below with the people who need help.

    1. _a_ habit disturbance groups
    2. _c_ general-purpose groups
    3. _d_ lifestyle organizations
    4. _b_ significant-other organizations
    5. _e_ physical handicap organizations

    a. Morgan's life is disrupted by his addiction to alcohol. He's looking for a self-help group of other alcoholics that he feels he can relate to.

    b. Morgan's wife, Paige, is very disturbed by her husband's drinking.

    c. A therapist at a community hospital wants to start a self-help group for persons who have recently dealt with the death of a loved one.

    d. Chris is sure that he has been discriminated against because of his obesity. He thinks a self-help group will help him deal with this problem and may even help change society's biased view.

    e. Pat is looking for a self-help organization for information about his cerebral palsy.

17-9	Can membership in self-help groups be therapeutic?

24. a. Why is it so difficult to empirically research the therapeutic effects of membership in a self-help group?

    b. Do active and involved members of self-help groups tend to experience mild, moderate or dramatic improvements as a result of membership?

17-10	What is psychosocial rehabilitation?

25. What two innovations, which occurred in the United States in the 1960's, were designed to enhance community based care of the mentally ill, but actually brought about a crisis of unemployment, homelessness, victimization and criminalization?

    a. *deinstitutionalization*

b. Mental Health Centers were built.

26. a. Describe psychosocial rehabilitation in your own words.

b. What three groups have worked together to advance psychosocial rehabilitation programs in the United States?

1. The National Alliance for the Mentally Ill

2. Self-help groups

3. Community-oriented mental health professionals

27. a. What is the goal of psychosocial rehabilitation?

b. Name the four components of psychosocial rehabilitation.

1. Help the person understand his disorder

2. Help the person identify & learn skills needed for community living.

3. Case management, to offer assistance in employment, housing, nutrition, finances, transportation, etc.

4. *Promote efforts to maintain a coalition among mental health professionals, family members + patients*

17-11   Can psychosocial rehabilitation effectively help severely mentally ill patients?

---

28. In your own words, briefly discuss what we have learned from research on the effectiveness of psychosocial rehabilitation. *Can teach individuals life + ~~self~~ self care skills, but performance does decline somewhat when the patient is out in the community. Relaps rates + other indicators of problems are ~~lower~~ lower for that patients who have gone through comprehensive psychosocial rehabilitation programs*

17-12   What is community psychology?

---

29. What four principles set community psychology apart from traditional clinical psychology?

a. *Community psychologists believe that behavior must be explained as an interaction of individuals + their environment.*

b. *Community psychologists believe intervention should take place in the settings where the client lives, works, or goes to school*

c. *Community psychologists make use of action research, which involves actual changes in the normal operation of social institutions*

d. *Community psychologists put a tremendous emphasis on prevention*

30. Match the following.

1. *C* tertiary prevention
2. *a* secondary prevention
3. *b* primary prevention

a.   also called selective prevention, focuses on people who are at risk for developing a disorder

b.   also called universal prevention, goals are to counteract risk factors and promote and reinforce protective measures as a way to prevent mental illness

c.   also called indicated prevention, focuses on people who show early signs of mental disorder

---

17-13   In what ways does community psychology attempt to promote the prevention of mental health problems?

---

31. What are five basic methods which are employed by community psychologists in the hope of preventing mental health problems?

a. help parents + children form strong, healthy attachments

b. teach children + adolescents effective cognitive + interpersonal skills, such as problem solving techniques, which will aid them in their development.

c. analyze environments which have a profound effect on development, such as families, schools, neighborhoods + the criminal justice system, +

d. then change them to make them more supportive reduce environmental stressors and/or help people cope more effectively w/ the major stressors they must endure.

e. promote empowerment by helping those who lack the confidence + ability to take control of their own lives to develop those characteristics.

17-14   How must prevention programs be designed if they are going to work?

32. Fill in the missing information in the table below.

COMMUNITY PSYCHOLOGISTS HAVE LEARNED THAT:	THEREFORE:
some especially damaging risk factors have widespread effects on human development. (see table 17.3)	these risk factors must receive the highest priority in prevention planning and programing.
most mental disorders are caused by a host of social, economic and psychological risk factors.	
risk factors tend to have cumulative effects; the longer they occur in people's lives the more serious are their consequences (the domino effect).	
certain risk factors are particularly dangerous during specific developmental stages.	
to be most effective, prevention programs need to take into account the cultural norms and values of the people they aim to help.	
the development of preventative interventions should be guided by risk factor theories that have been rigorously tested by research conducted in the natural environments where targeted disorders occur.	
primary prevention efforts introduce a special set of dilemmas and problems.	prevention scientists must often deal with unintended consequences, ethical questions and difficulties initiating programs and duplicating results of demonstration projects.

Test your understanding

1. Which of the following statements about self-help groups (SHG) is not true?
    a. Most SHG members usually have a well-defined problem or set of experiences.
    b. Self-help group meetings focus on exchanging information, providing feelings of togetherness and belonging and discussing mutual problems.
    c. Most self-help groups charge low or no fees. Their goal is to provide aid, not make a profit.
    d. Most self-help groups employ healthcare professionals in order to provide care and support for its members.

2. Alcoholics Anonymous and Gamblers Anonymous are examples of
    a. habit disturbance organizations.
    b. lifestyle organizations.
    c. significant-other organizations.
    d. physical handicap organizations.

3. Al-Anon is a self-help group for the relatives of alcoholics. It is an example of a
    a. habit disturbance organization.
    b. lifestyle organization.
    c. significant-other organization.
    d. physical handicap organization.

4. Self-help groups which address a wide range of difficulties are called
    a. habit disturbance organizations.
    b. lifestyle organizations.
    c. significant-other organizations.
    d. general-purpose groups.

5. Is it difficult to empirically research the therapeutic effects of self-help groups (SHG)?
    a. Yes, because most SHG are very secretive about their memberships and do not allow outsider researchers to attend group meetings.
    b. Yes, because the goals of most SHG are hard to precisely define.
    c. No, but empirical information is lacking because there has never been much interest by researchers into the effectiveness of SHG.
    d. No.

6. Active and involved members of self-help groups tend to experience _____ improvements as a result of membership.
    a. no
    b. mild
    c. moderate
    d. dramatic

7. The deinstitutionalization and the mental health center movements of the 1960's
    a. were the two most important factors which enhanced community based care of the mentally ill.
    b. were designed to enhance community based care of the mentally ill, but actually brought about a crisis of unemployment, homelessness, victimization and criminalization.
    c. were planned, but because of a lack of funding, never came about.
    d. did more than anything else to popularize the self-help care movement.

8. All of the following groups have worked together to advance psychosocial rehabilitation programs in the United States except
    a. the American Psychiatric Association.
    b. the National Alliance for the Mentally Ill.
    c. self-help groups.
    d. community-oriented mental health workers.

9. All of the following statements about the effectiveness of psychosocial rehabilitation services is true except
    a. psychosocial rehabilitation programs can teach a patient life and self-care skills.
    b. the performance of life and self-care behaviors decline somewhat when a patient goes into the community.
    c. relapse rates and other indicators of problems are lower for a patient who has gone through a comprehensive psychosocial rehabilitation program.
    d. psychosocial rehabilitation programs are so effective, that they may someday replace other forms of intervention.

10. Community psychology differs from traditional psychology in all of the following except
    a. community psychologists believe that behavior must be explained as an interaction between individuals and their environment.
    b. community psychologists believe that intervention should take place in the settings where the client lives, works or goes to school.
    c. community psychologists make use of action research which involves actual changes in the normal operation of social institutions.
    d. community psychologists put much less emphasis on prevention.

11. Tertiary prevention
    a. focuses on people who are at risk for developing a disorder.
    b. focuses on risk factors and promotes and reinforces protective measures as a way to prevent mental illness.
    c. focuses on people who show early signs of mental disorder.
    d. focuses on deinstitutionalization and mental health center programs as the main avenues of prevention.

12. Primary prevention
    a. focuses on people who are at risk for developing a disorder.
    b. focuses on risk factors and promotes and reinforces protective measures as a way to prevent mental illness.
    c. focuses on people who show early signs of mental disorder.
    d. focuses on deinstitutionalization and mental health center programs as the main avenues of prevention.

13. All of the following are methods employed by community psychologists in the hopes of preventing mental illness except
    a. building more mental health centers and community based mental hospitals.
    b. helping patients and children form stronger attachments.
    c. reducing environmental stressors.
    d. promoting empowerment.

14. Community psychologists have learned that
    a. all risk factors are basically of equal importance.
    b. most mental health problems are caused by one thing, stress.
    c. cultural norms and values are not significant factors in the effectiveness of prevention programs.
    d. certain risk factors are particularly dangerous during specific developmental stages.

15. Community psychologists working in primary prevention worry about the domino effect. This means that
    a. if parents are disordered, children will probably be disordered.
    b. if one person in a group has a disorder, others in that group will develop the same problems.
    c. risk factors have a cumulative effect, the longer they occur in people's lives, the greater the consequences.
    d. once funding is cut in one preventive program, other cuts soon follow.

Answers to test your understanding

1. d. (17-8)
2. a. (17-8)
3. c. (17-8)
4. d. (17-8)
5. b. (17-9)
6. c. (17-9)
7. b. (17-10)
8. a. (17-10)
9. d. (17-11)
10. d. (17-12)
11. c. (17-12)
12. b. (17-12)
13. a. (17-13)
14. d. (17-14)
15. c. (17-14)

When you have finished . . .

Explore the Web to find more information

The **American Association for Marriage and Family Therapy (AAMFT)** is a professional association comprised of marriage and family therapists from the United States, Canada and abroad.   Their URL is (**http://www.aamft.org/default.htm**). If you are looking for general information, WHAT IS MARRIAGE AND FAMILY THERAPY? is an especially informative link.

Internet Mental Health offers the article "Family Therapy," from The Harvard Medical School Mental Health Letter, Apr. (pt. I), May, 1988 (pt. II). (**http://www.mentalhealth.com/mag1/p5h-fam1.html**)

The **Alliance to Fight Eating Disorders (AFED)** is a good example of a self-help group and can be found at (http://www.fsci.umn.edu/~AAABL/default.htp).

You can explore the Web to find more information about psychosocial rehabilitation. The first document comes from **The World Health Organization**; the next three articles are from **Internet Mental Health**.

- "Psychosocial Rehabilitation: a Consensus Statement"
  (**http://www.who.ch/programmes/mnh/mnh/mnd/psr.htm**)

- "Preventing Relapse Through Therapeutic Partnership," *Prelapse Magazine*, No 3., April, 1996
  (**http://www.mentalhealth.com/mag1/pre-prev.html**)

- "An Innovative Approach to Vocational Rehabilitation," *Prelapse Magazine*, No 3., April, 1996
  (http://www.mentalhealth.com/mag1/pre-inno.html)

- "Putting the Mentally Ill to Work," The Harvard Mental Health Letter, July, 1996
  (http://www.mentalhealth.com/mag1/p5h-mh07.html)

The following articles from **Internet Mental Health** relate directly to the Controversy Box: "Can Violence Be Socially Inherited?" which is in this chapter.

- "The Fate of Violent Boys," The Harvard Mental Health Letter, May, 1995.
  (http://www.mentalhealth.com/mag1/fr51.html)

- "How the Cycle of Abuse Works," The Harvard Mental Health Letter, May, 1991.
  (http://www.mentalhealth.com/mag1/fr51.html)

CHAPTER 18
Legal and Ethical Issues
in Mental Disorders

Before you read . . .

Survey the chapter

Chapter 18 takes a different view of mental disorder than the preceding chapters in your text. Up to this point, the authors have mainly examined the effects of mental disorders on the diagnosed patient and the role of the therapist. In this chapter, the focus will shift to the human, ethical and legal issues surrounding the relationship between mental illness and the society at large.

Questions which will be addressed include: How can society strike a balance between the rights of a disturbed individual to control his or her own life and the rights of the general public who rely on nominative behavior from its members to function? What is the proper role of the government in the regulation and control of mental health services? In what ways do mental health professionals participate as experts in formal legal proceedings? Is it appropriate for them to do so? Should disturbed persons who commit crimes be judged innocent by reason of insanity?

As you read . . .

Ask questions

18-1   Thirty or forty years ago could a person be committed to a mental hospital against his or her will?

18-2   What long-ranging effects did the policy of deinstitutionalization have on the overall inpatient populations of mental hospitals and many of the individual patients themselves?

18-3   What are the commitment laws in use today?

18-4   Do mental health patients have the right to refuse treatment? Should mental health patients have the right to refuse treatment?

18-5   What are the legal rights of the mentally ill?

18-6   In what ways are mental health professionals regulated by the state?

18-7   Do therapists have a legal or ethical obligation to maintain confidentiality, even in situations where there is the potential of harm to others?

18-8   What kind of behaviors on the part of mental health workers constitute professional malpractice?

18-9   In what ways is mental health treatment regulated by economic controls?

18-10   In what ways is mental health treatment regulated by ethical standards?

18-11   In what ways do mental health professionals aid the legal system?

18-12   What is the insanity defense and how has it changed over time?

18-13   In what ways has the insanity defense been criticized?

18-14   In what ways has the insanity defense been revised?

After you read . . .

Review and explore the chapter

18-1   Thirty or forty years ago could a person be committed to a mental hospital against his or her will?

1. Throughout this text, you have read about the possible effects of mental illness on clients and the mental health professionals who work with them. In what ways do mental disorders affect the society in general?

2. What is therapeutic jurisprudence?

3. a. In your own words, briefly describe civil commitment.

b.   What was the traditional rationale which supported the use of civil commitment?

4.   Describe the social events which led up to the revision of civil commitment laws.

5.   The revisions of civil commitment laws in the late 1960's and 1970's required that before a person
could be involuntarily placed in a mental hospital, the state had to prove that four conditions existed.
What were they?

a.

b.

c.

d.

18-2   What long-ranging effects did the policy of deinstitutionalization have on the overall
inpatient populations of mental hospitals and many of the individual patients
themselves?

---

6.   In your own words, briefly describe the policy of deinstitutionalization.

7.   Although deinstitutionalization did a fine job of achieving the goal of dramatically lowering the
number of inpatients in mental hospitals, there are three reasons why most mental health professionals
believe that it did not meet its other goal of adequately shifting care from inpatient to outpatient

services. Discuss each of these three reasons.

a.

b.

c.

8. a.   As many as _____ (100,000 / 1,000,000) American citizens were homeless at the
         beginning of the 1990's and it is estimated that up to _____ (one-third / three-fourths) of
         them suffer from severe mental illness such as schizophrenia or bipolar disorder. As many as
         _____ (one-third / one-half) of these severely mentally ill homeless people are also alcohol
         or drug abusers.

    b.   Describe the disadvantages which are a common part of the homeless mentally ill's daily struggle
         for survival?

9. The National Institutes of Mental Health Task Force on Homelessness and Severe Mental Illness has
    proposed the creation of an integrated system of care for the homeless mentally ill. In your own
    words, briefly discuss each of the three components of this proposal.

    a.

    b.

    c.

10. What is meant by the concept of, the criminalization of the homeless mentally ill?

| 18-3 | What are the commitment laws in use today? |

11. By the 1980's, commitment laws began to change and reflect what is sometimes called the "thank-you theory" of commitment. Discuss the criteria for this involuntary commitment policy.

12. Match the following.

1. ____ commitment without court order
2. ____ commitment by court order
3. ____ outpatient commitment

a. most commonly used, especially in emergency situations

b. petition the court for psychiatric evaluation to determine if commitment criteria is satisfied

c. becoming more popular, especially when a patient is given a conditional release from a mental hospital

---

| 18-4 | Do mental health patients have the right to refuse treatment? Should mental health patients have the right to refuse treatment? |

13. a. What are the rules of implied consent?

b. Before the 1970's, were the rules of informed consent usually applied in cases of severe mental disorders?

14. a. Is the right to refuse treatment recognized in all states?

b. Has the Supreme Court ever held that the mentally ill have a constitutional right to refuse treatment?

15. a. Respond to the statement, "If mentally ill persons are allowed to refuse treatment, we will have hordes of unmedicated patients which will make wards chaotic, violent and dangerous."

b. Respond to the statement, "Patient refusal of treatment can result in increased costs."

18-5	What are the legal rights of the mentally ill?

16. Imagine that you are a lawyer. A person comes to you and asks the questions listed in the table below. How would you respond? Indicate the precedents which support your answers?

QUESTION	YOUR RESPONSE	PRECEDENT
A group of concerned neighbors comes before the city council demanding that a law be passed which will block the construction of a halfway house for recently discharged mental patients in their neighborhood. Can they do that?		Fair Housing Amendments Act of 1988 American with Disabilities Act of 1990 Cleburne Living Center v. City of Cleburne Texas
An inmate on death row, who displays the symptoms of paranoid schizophrenia, is judged legally insane. Can he be executed?		
In many states, mentally ill patients have the right to refuse treatment, but do they have the right to be treated and not merely confined?		

Can a nonviolent person who can live successfully in the community and has family support, be involuntarily confined in a mental institution?		
A mental patient who is not dangerous is put in restraints and food is withheld because she did not make her bed. Although this is obviously unethical, is it illegal?		

Test your understanding

1. What is therapeutic jurisprudence?
    a. the decision, by either a judge or jury, as to whether or not a nonviolent person should be committed involuntarily to an institution
    b. the decision, by either a judge or jury, as to whether or not an involuntarily committed patient should be released from an institution
    c. the consideration of the potential positive and negative therapeutic effects of legal rulings
    d. the social movement to deny institutionalized mental patients of their constitutional rights

2. What traditional rationale supported the use of civil commitment?
    a. *parens patriae*, "the country as parent"
    b. the United States Constitution
    c. "all for one - one for all"
    d. "out of sight, out of mind"

3. Which of the following was not a situation which led up to the revision of civil commitment laws?
    a. the social upheaval of the 1960's
    b. the civil-liberties movement
    c. The United States Supreme Court

    decision, Ford v. Wainwright
    d. the bias against psychiatry caused by its relative lack of success up to that point

4. The revisions of civil commitment laws in the late 1960's and 1970's required that before a person could be involuntarily committed to a mental hospital, all of the following conditions must exist except that
    a. the person is mentally ill.
    b. the person poses an imminent risk of danger to self or others.
    c. treatment is available.
    d. a family member or close friend gives written approval.

5. The policy of deinstitutionalization
    a. accomplished its goal of shifting care from outpatient to inpatient services.
    b. created a revolving door problem of numerous readmissions and short stays in inpatient settings.
    c. removed thousands of mentally ill homeless from the streets.
    d. dramatically lowered the number of persons in all types of inpatient services.

6. As many as _____ American citizens were homeless at the beginning of the 1990's and approximately _____ of them suffer from severe mental illness.
   a. 100,000, one-third
   b. 100,000, two-thirds
   c. one million, one-third
   d. one million, two-thirds

7. Which of the following is not part of the National Institutes of Mental Health Task Force on Homelessness and Severe Mental Illness' proposed system of care for the homeless mentally ill?
   a. assertive outreach
   b. safe havens
   c. integrated care and support services
   d. managed care system approach

8. What is meant by the concept of the "criminalization of the homeless mentally ill"?
   a. The homeless mentally ill are often arrested and jailed due to their disturbed behavior, lack of acceptance by society and/or police trying to avoid the red tape involved in hospitalization.
   b. An increasing number of communities have passed laws attempting to bar the homeless mentally ill from sleeping on their streets.
   c. New laws make homelessness a criteria for involuntary commitment to mental hospitals.
   d. Once in the legal system, persons who are homeless and mentally ill are incarcerated in prisons at a significantly higher rate than are persons in the general population.

9. Many states in the 1980's changed their commitment laws to reflect the idea that individual rights should not be placed above alleviation of suffering. This is sometimes referred to as
   a. the parental theory of commitment.
   b. the thank-you theory of commitment.

   c. the Big Brother theory of commitment.
   d. the diminishment of suffering / individual rights ratio.

10. Which of the following types of commitment in use today is increasing in popularity, especially when a patient is given a conditional release from a mental hospital?
   a. commitment without court order
   b. commitment with court order
   c. outpatient commitment
   d. relapse prevention commitment, with or without court order

11. Has the Supreme Court ever held that the mentally ill have a constitutional right to refuse treatment?
   a. Yes. The court has held that this is true in all cases.
   b. Yes. The court has held that this is true, but only in cases of voluntary commitment.
   c. No. In fact, no federal or state law recognizes the right of mental patients to refuse treatment.
   d. No. In fact, in some states mental patients can be ordered to comply with treatment that a professional deems necessary.

12. Does federal law prohibit housing discrimination against people with mental disorders and retardation?
   a. No. Federal laws concerning this have never been passed because of the potential political problems.
   b. No. Laws prohibiting housing discrimination were struck down as unconstitutional in 1975.
   c. Yes. This is included in the Fair Housing Act of 1988 and the Americans with Disabilities Act.
   d. Yes. This is covered in the Fair and Equal Access to Housing mandates of 1980, 1982 and 1991.

13. The execution of insane prisoners
    a. is unconstitutional and, therefore, never occurs in this country.
    b. is unconstitutional, but probably still occurs in this country.
    c. is a matter of individual state law. It is prohibited in some states and allowed in others.
    d. is a matter of state law. No state has allowed it since 1963.

14. A friend tells you that legally, the minimal amount of care that a mental hospital needs to provide is safe and humane confinement.
    a. Your friend is correct. The legal precedent is Rouse v. Cameron.
    b. Your friend is correct. The legal precedent is the Americans with Disabilities Act.
    c. Your friend is wrong. Although ethical rules may apply, no law states that the confinement needs to be safe or humane.
    d. Your friend is wrong. Patients have a constitutional right to safe and humane confinement, as well as a legal right to receive treatment.

15. Does the need to treat a mental disorder provide the legal justification for the involuntary commitment of a nonviolent person, even if that person can function in the community with family support?
    a. no
    b. yes, in all cases
    c. yes, in Tennessee, Illinois and Colorado
    d. yes, in Ohio, Nebraska and Missouri

Answers to test your understanding

1. c. (18-1)
2. a. (18-1)
3. c. (18-1)
4. d. (18-1)
5. b. (18-2)
6. c. (18-2)
7. d. (18-2)
8. a. (18-3)
9. b. (18-3)
10. c. (18-3)
11. d. (18-4)
12. c. (18-5)
13. b. (18-5)
14. d. (18-5)
15. a. (18-5)

18-6   In what ways are mental health professionals regulated by the state?

17. Match the following.

1. ____ certification laws
2. ____ licensure laws
3. ____ privilege
4. ____ confidentiality

    a. a legal requirement which protects certain persons from public disclosure in court

b. restricts the use of a professional title to people who have met certain requirements for education, practical training and supervised experience

c. an ethical obligation that therapists do not disclose communications between their clients and themselves

d. restricts the use of a professional title to people who have met certain requirements for education, practical training and supervised experience, as well as restricting the practice of a given profession

---

18-7   Do therapists have a legal or ethical obligation to maintain confidentiality, even in situations where there is the potential of harm to others?

---

18. Describe five situations where a therapist may be forced to breach confidentiality.

a.

b.

c.

d.

e.

19. a.   In your own words, briefly discuss the Tarasoff decision.

b.   At the time of the Tarasoff decision, many psychotherapists feared that the impact would be antitherapeutic. Why?

c.   What was the actual impact of the Tarasoff decision?

18-8   What kind of behaviors on the part of mental health workers constitute professional malpractice?

20. In order to prove a claim of professional malpractice, four elements must be established. Discuss each of them below.

a.

b.

c.

d.

21. a.   Even though sexual intimacy in a therapeutic relationship is unethical and can result in malpractice claims, what percentage of mental health workers report that they have been sexually intimate with a client?

b.   Discuss five reasons that sexual contact between therapist and client is unethical?

1.

2.

3.

4.

5.

c.   Is sexual contact between a therapist and a former client prohibited by the APA?

22. In your own words, briefly describe how repressed memory therapy can result in malpractice suits.

| 18-9 | In what ways is mental health treatment regulated by economic controls? |

23. a.   In your own words, briefly describe how intervention is delivered in a managed care system.

b.   Why do many therapists oppose economic incentives inherent in a managed care system?

18-10   In what ways is mental health treatment regulated by ethical standards?

24. a.   How does the text define ethical standards?

b.   What types of behaviors are covered by the APA's Code of Ethical Principles of Psychologists and Code of Conduct.

18-11   In what ways do mental health professionals aid the legal system?

25. List and briefly discuss the four basic services which mental health workers generally provide to the legal system.

a.

b.

c.

d.

26. a.   What is forensic psychology and forensic psychiatry?

b.   What are three reasons why expert testimony by mental health professionals is used so
     frequently?

     1.

     2.

     3.

27. What criteria are used to decide if a defendant is considered incompetent to stand trial?

18-12	What is the insanity defense and how has it changed over time?

28. Fill in the missing information.

INSANITY STANDARD	DATE	SUMMARY
McNaughton Rule		
Durham Rule		
American Law Institute (ALI) Rule		

> 18-13   In what ways has the insanity defense been criticized?

29. Are the following statements about the insanity defense true or false? If the statement is false, correct it by making the appropriate changes.

    a.   Across the United States, approximately 15-17 percent of all criminal cases involve a finding of NGRI.

    b.   The major problem with the NGRI verdict is that the majority of defendants go completely free within one year.

    c.   It is unclear if hospital confinements and treatment have any clear benefits for defendants found NGRI, because research results have been mixed.

    d.   Studies show that the insanity defense is so costly that the average defendant cannot afford to use it.

    e.   Questions about the testimony of mental health experts have been raised concerning the ability of experts to be accurate, the influence they may exert on the outcome of the trial and the possible damage to the public's confidence in the behavioral sciences.

> 18-14   In what ways has the insanity defense been revised?

30. In your own words, briefly discuss each of the following reforms introduced in insanity defense rules.

    a.   the guilty, but mentally ill verdict

b.   the Insanity Defense Reform Act

c.   abolition of the insanity defense

Test your understanding

1.   Licensure laws
    a.   are legal requirements which protect certain persons from public disclosure in court.
    b.   restrict the use of a professional title to people who have met certain requirements.
    c.   deal with ethical obligations that therapists do not disclose communications between their clients and themselves.
    d.   restrict both the use of a professional title to people who have met certain requirements and the practice of a given profession.

2.   Confidentiality refers to
    a.   legal requirements which protect certain persons from public disclosure in court.
    b.   the restriction of the use of a professional title to people who have met certain requirements.
    c.   ethical obligations that therapists do not disclose communications between their clients and themselves.
    d.   the restrictions on both the use of a professional title to people who have met certain requirements and the practice of a given profession.

3.   Which of the following is not a situation in which a therapist may be forced to breach confidentiality?

    a.   The therapist believes that the client needs to be involuntarily committed.
    b.   The therapist learns that the client is abusing other people.
    c.   The client raises the issue of his or her mental condition and the therapist must testify in court.
    d.   The therapist is contacted by a biological child of the client with a request for genetic counseling.

4.   The Tarasoff decision was a landmark case involving the responsibility of therapists to
    a.   report sexual conduct between fellow therapists and clients.
    b.   take steps to protect any potential victims of their dangerous clients.
    c.   report recovered memories of sexual abuse.
    d.   refuse to follow a court order, if doing so would hinder the client's therapeutic progress.

5.   Which of the following is not one of the four elements that must be established in order to prove a claim of malpractice?
    a.   A professional relationship had to exist between the client and therapist.
    b.   The client had to have suffered harm.
    c.   The therapist had to have intentionally set out to harm the client.
    d.   The harm suffered by the client was caused by the therapist's negligence.

6. What percentage of mental health workers report that they have been sexually intimate with a client?
    a. less than 1/10 of 1 percent
    b. 1 percent
    c. 5-8 percent
    d. 15 percent

7. One statement about the existence and cause of repressed memories on which almost all professionals in the behavioral sciences would agree, is
    a. this is a hotly debated topic.
    b. repressed memories are nothing more than beliefs which have been intentionally planted by therapists.
    c. repressed memories are nothing more than beliefs which have been unintentionally planted by well-meaning therapists.
    d. repressed memories are accurate recollections of actual events.

8. Which two of the following are reasons why many therapists are opposed to managed care systems (MCS)?
    a. MCS are not very cost effective.
    b. MCS are so cost effective, the therapist's income is often cut by half.
    c. There is an incentive to put profit above quality of care.
    d. Treatment decisions are often made by a case manager who is not a mental health professional.

9. The professional behaviors of members of the American Psychological Association are
    a. governed by the Code of Ethical Principles of Psychologists and Code of Conduct.
    b. governed by the DSM-IV Ethics Manual.
    c. governed by the Therapist's Guide to Ethical Behavior and Appropriate Conduct, third edition-revised.
    d. not subject to a professional code of ethics.

10. _____ and _____ are specialty fields which apply mental health knowledge to questions about individuals involved in legal proceedings.
    a. therapeutic jurisprudence - legal psychology
    b. behavioral criminal justice - legal psychiatry
    c. forensic psychology - forensic psychiatry
    d. criminal psychiatry - criminal psychology

11. In order to be judged incompetent to stand trial, a defendant must, because of his or her mental disorder, meet all of the following criteria except he or she must
    a. be unable to understand the nature of the trial proceedings.
    b. be unable to participate meaningfully in his or her own defense.
    c. be unable to consult with his or her attorney.
    d. be unable to emotionally cope with the stress of a criminal trial.

12. In 1843, which of the following set the original standard for finding a person not guilty by reason of insanity?
    a. the McNaughton Rule
    b. the Durham Rule
    c. the American Law Institute Rule
    d. the Americans with Disabilities Act

13. About what percentage of all criminal cases end in a finding of not guilty by reason of insanity?
    a. fewer than 1 percent
    b. 5-8 percent
    c. 10 percent
    d. 22 percent

14. Which of the following statements about the not guilty by reason of insanity (NGRI) plea is not true?
    a.   Defendants found NGRI seldom go completely free.
    b.   It is unclear if hospital confinements and treatment have any clear benefits for defendants found NGRI, because research results have been mixed.
    c.   Studies show that the insanity defense is so costly that the average defendant cannot afford to use it.
    d.   Questions about the testimony of mental health experts in NGRI cases have been raised concerning the ability of experts to be accurate.

15. Which of the following is not an attempt to reform insanity defense rules?
    a.   the guilty, but mentally ill verdict
    b.   the Insanity Defense Reform Act
    c.   section four of the Americans with Disabilities Act
    d.   abolition of insanity defense

Answers to test your understanding

1.   d.   (18-6)
2.   c.   (18-6)
3.   d.   (18-7)
4.   b.   (18-7)
5.   c.   (18-8)
6.   c.   (18-8)
7.   a.   (18-8)
8.   c. d. (18-9)
9.   a.   (18-10)
10. c.   (18-11)
11. d.   (18-11)
12. a.   (18-12)
13. a.   (18-13)
14. c.   (18-13)
15. c.   (18-14)

When you have finished . . .

Explore the Web to find more information

An overview of many of the issues raised in this chapter can be found in the **World Health Organization** document, "Mental Health Care Law: Ten Basic Principles." You can find it by going to (**http://www.who.ch/programmes/mnh/mnh/mnd/legal.htm**).

If you are looking for more information on involuntary commitment, you may be interested in the article, "What Are the Current Standards for Involuntary Commitment to a Mental Hospital?" from The Harvard Mental Health Letter, May, 1991. It is provided by **Internet Mental Health**. It can be accessed at (**http://www.mentalhealth.com/mag1/p5h-mh05.html**).

If you are looking for information on deinstitutionalization or the homeless mentally ill these articles may interest you. They are also provided by **Internet Mental Health**.

- "Deinstitutionalization: What Will It Really Cost?" by John Martin B.A., M.T.S., M.A., *Schizophrenia Digest*, April, 1995. (**http://www.mentalhealth.com/mag1/p51-sc02.html**)

- "The Prevalence of Homelessness," The Harvard Mental Health Letter, April, 1996. (**http://www.mentalhealth.com/mag1/p5h-hom5.html**)

- "Mental Illness and Homelessness," The Harvard Mental Health Letter, July, (Part I), August, 1990 (Part II). (**http://www.mentalhealth.com/mag1/p5h-hom4.html**)

- "Schizophrenia and Homelessness," *Prelapse Magazine*, No. 2, September, 1995. (**http://www.mentalhealth.com/mag1/pre-hom1.html**)

The complete text of "The Americans With Disabilities Act of 1990," is available through the **United States Department of Justice** at (**http://gopher.usdoj.gov/crt/ada/statute.html**).

The American Psychological Association provides an interesting article, "The Americans With Disabilities Act and How It Affects Psychologists," at (**http://www.apa.org/pi/act.html**).

Here are several links which deal with some of the questions of professional ethics posed in this chapter. The first two are articles provided by **Internet Mental Health**.

- "Confidentiality in Mental Health Treatment," The Harvard Medical School Mental Health Letter, February, 1988. (**http://www.mentalhealth.com/mag1/p5h-cfd1.html**)

- "Can Therapists be Sued for Recovered Memories?", The Harvard Mental Health Letter, April, 1996. (**http://www.mentalhealth.com/mag1/p5h-mem1.html**)

- If you are interested in the discussion of recovered memory, "Questions and Answers about Memories of Childhood Abuse," an article from the **American Psychological Association**, is located at (**http://www.apa.org/pubinfo/mem.html**).

- "If Sex Enters Into the Therapy Relationship," a Public Interest Directorate, published by the **The American Psychological Association**, can be found at (**http://www.apa.org/pi/therapy.html**).

The complete text of **The American Psychological Association's** "Ethical Principles of Psychologists and Code of Conduct," is available through the APA at (**http://www.apa.org/ethics/code.html**).

Chapter 1 - Abnormal Behavior: Past and Present Perspectives

1. a disturbance of an individual's behavioral, psychological, or physical functioning that is not culturally expected and that leads to psychological distress, behavioral disability or impaired overall functioning

2.

TIME PERIOD/ CULTURE	HOW DID THEY EXPLAIN?	HOW DID THEY RESPOND?
Prehistoric	evil spirit / supernatural forces	trephining
Ancient Chinese, Egyptian, Hebrew	evil spirit / supernatural forces	prayer, faith healing, rest, exercise, diet
Greek	biological factors, humor imbalance	medicine, diet, laxatives and purgatives to restore balance
Roman	humors, role of brain	medicine, diet, physical therapy
Chinese (Taoism)	imbalance of yin and yang	moderation in behavior, openness to nature's healing forces

3. 1. b.
   2. a.
   3. g.
   4. e.
   5. f.
   6. c.
   7. h.
   8. d.
4. develop, treat
5. An hypothesis is an educated prediction about how two or more variables are related. They are tested by empirical methods. As evidence accumulates, scientists organize their explanations into theories, which are more generalized sets of propositions used to predict and explain a phenomenon.
6. a. A correlation is a statistical measure of the degree to which one variable is related to another.
   b. Two variables are positively correlated when they change together in the same direction.
   c. Two variables are negatively correlated when they move in opposite directions.
7. An experiment. Correlations cannot establish a causal relationship between two variables.
8. 1. a.
   2. d.
   3. h.
   4. e.
   5. f.
   6. g.
   7. c.
   8. b.
9. The basic assumption is that the nervous system controls all thought and behavior, both normal and abnormal.

10. symptoms, etiological
11. 1. b.
    2. e.
    3. f.
    4. c.
    5. a.
    6. d.
12.

BRAIN AREA	BRAIN STRUCTURE	FUNCTION
Hindbrain	medulla	breathing, swallowing, heart rate, blood pressure
	reticular formation	arousal, attention, sleep-wakefulness cycles
	cerebellum	balance, posture, fine motor functions
Midbrain		gross movement, coordination and responsiveness to sensory and rewarding stimuli
Forebrain	thalamus	relay of sensory stimuli
	hypothalamus	hunger, thirst, sex drive
	limbic system	emotion, memory
Cerebrum	cerebral cortex	higher level cognitive processes

13. a. They are chemicals which carry messages between neurons in the brain and nervous system.
    b. Neurotransmitters either stimulate or inhibit the firing of neurons. They are the basis for nervous system communication.
    c. Drugs that alter the levels or activity of neurotransmitters can produce complex psychological and behavioral effects which can possibly be therapeutic.
14. nucleotides, chromosomes, proteins, genotype, phenotype
15. a. examine the pattern of disorder in members of the same family
    b. study traits and disorders in persons who were separated from their biological parents
    c. compare characteristics of twins who were separated near birth and raised in different environments
16. a. no
    b. no
    c. yes
17. 1. c.
    2. a.
    3. d.
    4. b.
18. Your answers should include the following:
    a. (first year) The main source of pleasure is oral gratification.
    b. (second year) The focus is on elimination and retention of feces. Toilet training is important.
    c. (age 3 -4) The focus is on genitals. For boys, sexual desire is for his mother (Oedipal complex). For girls, the focus is inferiority (penis envy).
    d. (age 5- adolescence) As turmoil subsides, focus shifts to

same-sex friendships.

  e.   (adolescence) The focus is on genital pleasure, which fuses with love relationships.

19. a.   To help the client gain insight into the unconscious origins of his or her behavior.

    b.   1.   free association - Client responds to words or phrases with whatever comes into their mind without trying to control it

         2.   interpretation - dreams, slips of the tongue, everyday mistakes are examined to reveal hidden motives

         3.   transference - by reliving past emotional reactions clients will recognize their importance and conflicts will be minimized

20. a.   Your answer should include the idea that all specific behaviors, whether normal or abnormal are shaped by the person's experiences.

    b.   1.   the relationship between behavior and its consequences

         2.   the association which develops between environmental stimuli and behavioral responses

         3.   behavior is affected not only by environmental consequences, but also by the thoughts and expectations people use to process and understand information about their lives

21. 1.   a.
     2.   e.
     3.   c.
     4.   f.
     5.   d.
     6.   b.

22. an unconditioned, an unconditioned
a neutral
a conditioned, a conditioned

23. Your answer should include the idea that the goal of behavior therapy is to decrease maladaptive behaviors and increase adaptive ones by using the basic laws of learning theory.

24. a.   learning occurs as a result of the way people process information about the world, how they pay attention to, form perceptions of, think about, and remember stimuli

    b.   1.   often behavior is learned as a result of observing other people's behavior and its consequences

         2.   the probability that a behavior will occur depends on the person's expectations of the outcome of that behavior

         3.   our interpretations of events are influenced by how we evaluate our behavior and the behavior of others

         4.   expectations for behavior and other events which affect our experience of and interpretation of that event

         5.   negative and unrealistic expectancies for behavior and the outcome of events

25. irrational or distorted thinking

26. Your answer should include the idea that human behavior is determined by each person's unique perception of the world at any given moment.

27. a.   People have an innate drive toward personal growth (self-actualization). All behavior is understandable as a reflection of the individual's efforts toward growth, his or her self-concept and his or her perception of the world. Incongruence and unhealthy conditions of worth are barriers toward personal growth

    b.   Unmet needs block a person's natural motivation to attain self-actualization.

28. a.   The therapeutic relationship must be free of conditions of worth.

    b.   helping persons overcome the obstacles that block the

natural process of growth and fulfillment

29. a.   People interact easily and smoothly as they negotiate their complementary needs.

    b.   People use problematic interpersonal ploys to get what they want. This can destroy smooth patterns of interaction, hurt the relationship and cause unhappiness and further problems

30. helping people give up problematic interpersonal styles and develop more flexible, less extreme ways of relating to others

31. internal, external

32. a.   cultural hardships such as poverty, racism, inferior education, unemployment and social changes put people at a greater risk for behavioral disorders

    b.   a higher rate of some disorders at lower socioeconomic levels is due to the fact that those lower socioeconomic levels contain a disproportionately high number of persons with behavior problems

    c.   standards and definitions of abnormal behavior vary widely in different places and for different groups

    d.   mental disorders are simply labels placed on behaviors that are problematic at that time and for that particular population

33. Your answer should include the idea that behavioral disorders result from the combination of a diathesis (predisposition for that disorder) and a stressor (any event which causes stress, and therefore triggers the development of the predisposed problem).

34. Because of the emphasis on the interaction of individual characteristics with changing environments, effective treatment must include a combination of techniques to deal with all aspects of the dynamic situation.

Chapter 2 - Assessment and Diagnosis

1. It is difficult because there are many different theoretical perspectives that need to be taken into account - religious, medical, psychological, and sociocultural.

2. a.   Your answer should include the idea that persons who act in ways which differ from the definitions of what is appropriate behavior for a group are often labeled as deviant or abnormal.

    b.   rare, negative

    c.   1.   It ignores characteristics which are not rare, but still problematic.

         2.   There is no agreed upon definition as to how rare a condition must be in order to qualify it as a disorder.

         3.   Just because a behavior is expected and common in a group, doesn't necessarily mean that it is healthy.

3. a.   Your answer should include the idea that a mental disorder exists if a behavior is treated by a mental health professional.

    b.   the onset and frequency of disorders in certain populations.

    c.   simplicity

    d.   1.   not everyone who consults a clinician n is suffering symptoms

         2.   not all persons suffering symptoms have access to professional help

4. a.   Your answer should include the idea that personal distress and unhappiness is commonly seen in mental disorders and is often the reason people to seek treatment.

    b.   1.   Distress alone cannot define disorder, in fact it is commonly seen at times in all people.

2.   There is often no distinction between acute distress and distress that is chronic, intense and not related to external events.

3.   Some persons with patterns of problematic behavior, such as personality disorders, show little or no distress.

5.   a.   Your answer should include the idea that a disorder exists, if a behavior which results from some physical or psychological breakdown, causes a problem in living.

b.   It is an example of dysfunction, because there is a physical breakdown in brain function which affects memory.

c.   It is an example of harm, because becoming lost is a negative result of the brain dysfunction related to the Alzheimer's disease.

d.   1.   It is difficult to define specific limits which describe when an impairment becomes a dysfunction.

2.   Criteria for judging dysfunction and harm may vary from culture to culture.

3.   It is difficult to define specific limits which describe when an impairment becomes a harm which requires treatment and not just an annoyance which requires patience.

e.   Yes. It is the most workable and least arbitrary definition.

6.   a.   Assessment, diagnose

b.   1.   First, the clinician gathers assessment information.

2.   Next, he or she will organize and process this information into a description of the person that the clinician is assessing.

3.   Finally, the clinician will compare this description to what is known about various disorders.

7.   1.   c.
     2.   b.
     3.   d.
     4.   a.

8.   1.   c.
     2.   a.
     3.   d.
     4.   b.
     5.   e.

9.   1.   a.
     2.   b.
     3.   d.
     4.   f.
     5.   e.
     6.   c.

10. a.   They are documents associated with important events in a person's life.

b.   no

11. 1.   b.
     2.   a.
     3.   c.
     4.   d.

12. structured, superior, less

13. 1.   d.
     2.   f.
     2.   c.
     4.   b.
     5.   a.
     6.   e.
     7.   g.
     8.   h.

14. It is the most widely used objective personality test.

15. 1.   b.
     2.   d.
     3.   c.
     4.   e.

5.   f.
6.   a.

16. a.   internal changes in physical structure and function which are neither observable or reportable by clients themselves

b.   No. CAT scans only provide images of brain structure, not function. The appropriate choice would be PET scans or MRI.

17. a.   Diagnostic and Statistical Manual of Mental Disorders (I denotes first edition - 1952, II denotes second edition - 1968, III denotes third edition - 1980, III-R denotes third edition revised - 1987)

b.   American Psychiatric Association

c.   because there were many different and conflicting systems in use

18. a.   provided specific and clear diagnostic criteria, avoided theoretical assumptions about disorders, introduced multiaxial classification

b.   criteria still vague, inadequate attention to diversity issues, problems with construct validity

19. It was based on empirical research done in field trials.

20.

DSM AXIS	ATTRIBUTES DESCRIBED ON THAT AXIS
Axis I	sixteen groupings of major mental disorders
Axis II	ten personality disorders
Axis III	medical conditions relevant to disorder
Axis IV	measure of the stress a person has been under in the last year
Axis V	measure of overall level of functioning

21. 1.   b.
     2.   c.
     3.   a.
     4.   e.
     5.   d.

22. 1.   b.
     2.   a.
     3.   d.
     4.   c.
     5.   e.

23. 1.   e.
     2.   d.
     3.   c.
     4.   b.
     5.   a.
     6.   f.

24. Yes. Different disorders can result from the same cause, one disorder can lead to the development of another disorder and different disorders often share the same criteria. It is called co-morbidity.

25. Your answers should include the ideas that:

a.   labeling can have a negative effect by distorting how a person is looked at by others and by themselves (self-fulfilling process).

b.   symptoms of disorder can not fit in neat packages that are always easy to differentiate from "normal" behavior.

c.   in order to enhance reliability, the diagnostic criteria are so simple and specific that the true nature of some disorders may have been lost.

d.   DSM labels imply that mental disorders are more influenced by individual internal factors than by social factors.

26. Your answers should include the ideas that:
   a. the diagnosis may be influenced by the type of insurance benefits available for the patient.
   b. a clinician who is interested in or specializes in a specific area may possible bias the diagnosis toward that area.
   c. primary care physicians often under-diagnose mental disorders.
27. 1. a.
    2. c.
    3. b.
28. a. Most psychological tests were developed and normed on white populations.
    b. 1. Differences between groups may be caused by diversity in language, culture, etc., not by what the test is designed to measure.
       2. Findings relevant to one group may not be valid for another group.
29. Your answer should include the idea that the cultural background of a person may affect their specific definition of what constitutes a problem, as well as their willingness and ability to relate their concerns to the clinician.
30. prevalence, incidence
31. a. The lifetime prevalence for a major mental disorder is 32 percent.
    b. The lifetime prevalence of mental disorders is frequently related to demographic or social variables.
    c. The most common disorders are phobias and alcohol abuse, followed by generalized anxiety disorder, major depression and drug abuse or dependence.
    d. Almost 40 percent of persons were symptom free during the previous year.
    e. Less than one-fifth of persons with mental disorders report receiving recent treatment. In those cases, the treatment was most often rendered by general physicians.
    f. Co-morbidity of mental disorders is common.
    g. The average age for noticing the first symptoms is 16.

Chapter 3 - Disorders of Infancy, Childhood, and Adolescence

1. a. the increased use of prospective longitudinal studies as opposed to retrospective methods
   b. advances in classification and measurement of children's behaviors
2. a. behavioral patterns occurring between infancy to adolescence on which further developmental adjustment rests
   b. Examples can include: forming attachments, attaining self-reliance, academic competence or healthy separation from the family.
   c A child's failure to effectively adjust to an early developmental task will affect his or her capacity to handle later tasks successfully.
3. Early problems in completing a developmental task may increase the likelihood of later problems.
4. a. It is a laboratory assessment technique which examines infant-parent attachment.
   b. Infants show moderate separation distress and a strong approach to parent during reunions.
   c. Patterns include: minimal separation distress or excessive separation distress which is not lessened by parent's return and contradictory, undirected or confused behaviors during reunion.

d. Insecure
5. a. Your answer should include the idea that disorders have clear symptomatic boundaries that distinguish normal behavior from abnormal behavior, as well as one disorder from another. People either "fit" into a description or they don't.
   b. the DSM-IV
6. a. Your answer should include the idea that abnormal behavior cannot accurately be described in black and white categories. Behavior should be described in ways that reflect different degrees.
   b. Externalizing problems are undercontrolled and excessive undesirable behavior patterns. They are subdivided into aggressive and delinquent.
   c. Internalizing problems are overcontrolled deficits in desired behavior. They are subdivided into withdrawn, somatic (physical) complaints and anxious/depressed.
7. the most, 60-70
8. externalizing
9. a. very poor control over emotions
   b. extremely noncompliant and argumentative with parents and teachers
   c. repeated conflicts with peers
   d. blaming others for mistakes
10. The oppositional behavior is producing impairment in social relations, school performance or other aspects of functioning.
11. a. There is a good chance that preschoolers will continue to engage in troublesome behavior. About one-third will have significant problems at age nine. The majority of grade schoolers will show later conduct problems, aggression and antisocial behaviors.
    b. problems occur in more than one setting; aggression and hyperactivity; co-occur with ODD; lying and stealing co-occur with arguing and aggression; family stress
12. To diagnose conduct disorder, the child must show behaviors which are potentially harmful to themselves, others or property.
13.

CATEGORY	SUMMARY OF BEHAVIORS
Aggression to people and animals	bullies and threatens others, initiates and uses weapon in fights, cruelty to others and animals, stealing, forcing someone into sexual activity
Destruction of property	setting fires or in other ways destroying property intentionally
Deceitfulness or theft	lies often, theft without confronting victim, breaking into houses
Serious violation of rules	running away, truancy

14. more, more
15. a. Your answer should include the idea that even though human studies are inconclusive, animal studies suggest a correlation between aggression and high levels of testosterone.
    b. Your answer should include the idea that low levels of serotonin are associated with high levels of aggression.
    c. Your answer should include the idea that children with CD have lower resting heart rates which may indicate less capacity for the fear response which mediates risk-taking behavior.
16. a. Your answer should include the idea that deficits in cognitive abilities correlate with increased rates of CD, especially early onset type.

b. Your answer should include the idea that coercive cycles of aggression, extreme criticism, frequent commands and lack of warmth correlate with high levels of CD.

c. Your answer should include the idea that environmental issues such as substance abuse, poverty and stress correlate with higher rates of CD.

d. Your answer should include the idea that children with CD are less likely to possess the cognitive skills necessary to respond to problems in nonaggressive ways.

17. a. It is designed to teach parents to interact effectively with their children.

    b. Yes, in some cases it leads to significant changes in the child's behavior.

    c. 1. There is often no improvement in behavior at school or other environments.

      2. It is less effective with parents who are under high stress or lack effective parenting skills.

      3. There is no strong long-term effect on early onset CD.

18. a. attempt to change child's perceptual inaccuracies, biased expectations of hostility, limited awareness of non-aggressive problem solving skills and language deficits

    b. can increase social skills and reduce disruptive behavior in the short-term

19. a. inattention; example: difficulty listening to teacher at school

    b. hyperactivity; example: fidgets at desk

    c. impulsivity; example: blurts out answers, interrupts

20. ADHD symptoms must cause significant impairment in two or more settings.

21. 3-5, Boys, lower

22. a. ADHD-H
    b. ADHD-I
    c. ADHD-H
    d. ADHD-I
    e. ADHD-I
    f. ADHD-H

23. Seventy percent of elementary school-age children diagnosed with ADHD still meet DSM criteria by mid-adolescence. About half will also meet criteria for CD. Many adults will continue to meet ADHD criteria in their twenties and thirties, with increased co-morbidity with substance abuse and antisocial behavior.

24. a. Low birth weight, oxygen deprivation and fetal alcohol syndrome may be correlated with ADHD.

    b. The incidence of ADHD among relatives is much higher than in the general population.

    c. Abnormally low RAS activity may create the need for extra stimulation.

    d. ADHD children may have smaller and/or lower functioning frontal lobes, which control executive functions such as planning and carrying out goal-directed behaviors.

25. parental intrusiveness and overstimulation

26. a. They increase the activity of norepinephrine and dopamine which enhances the ability to focus and reduces ADHD symptoms.

    b. Yes, about 75 percent show a positive response.

    c. short lasting effects and rebound effect

27. behavior management and cognitive-behavioral interventions

28. similar to

29. a. yes

    b. The anxiety must be persistent and interfere significantly with functioning.

30. a. observable behaviors (avoidance, etc.)

    b. physiological arousal (upset stomach, sweating, etc.)

    c. cognition (constant worry)

31.

BEHAVIORS ASSOCIATED WITH SAD	
1.	child is clingy and dependent on adults, demanding help for even the simplest tasks
2.	worry about parents getting sick or injured
3.	excessive fear of being left alone
4.	nightmares
5.	refusal to go to school
6.	can't tolerate leaving parents for even a few hours
7.	physical complaints

32. School refusal in social phobia is the result of the fear of embarrassment or humiliation. In specific phobia it is the result of fear of a single stimulus, such as a specific school activity. In SAD it is related to the fear of being away from the parent.

33. inhibition

34. a. Your answer should include the idea that inhibited and anxious children have heightened signs of physical arousal, such as accelerated heart rate and higher levels of norepinephrine.

    b. Your answer should include the idea that environmental stressors, the "match" between the child's temperament and the parent's style of parenting and social relationships which either encourage or discourage fearful behavior, may play a role in the development of separation anxiety disorder.

    c. Your answer should include the idea that anxious children expect bad things to happen, blame themselves for problems and exaggerate the threatening aspects of unfamiliar situations.

35. Your answer should include the idea that the child learns anxiety reducing techniques and applies them during gradual exposure to fearful situations involving separation.

36. Your answer should include the idea that cognitive restructuring, coping skills training and self-reinforcement for statements of positive self-worth are used in cognitive therapy.

37. Your answer should include the idea that the use of antidepressants have played a limited role in the treatment of separation anxiety disorder.

38.

SYMPTOM CATEGORY	SPECIFIC BEHAVIORS
Mood / Negative feelings	irritability, sadness, hopelessness
Health	complaints of physical ailments
View of self / environment	low self-esteem, interpret situations negatively
Relationships with others	problems making and keeping friends
Self-destructive tendencies	suicidal thoughts and attempts, substance abuse, reckless play, reckless driving

39. a. Your answer should include the idea that children who are at risk for depression may show the same cerebral asymmetry that is seen in depressed adults.
    b. Your answer should include the idea that children of depressed parents have significantly higher rates of depression themselves.
    c. Depressed children are more likely to use avoidant, aggressive or passive behaviors when experiencing sadness.
40. a. Recent studies question the effectiveness of tricyclic antidepressants and they can cause negative side effects.
    b. Cognitive-behavioral treatments such as cognitive restructuring, coping skills training and self-reinforcement.
41. a. AN
    b. BN
    c. AN
    d. BN
    e. BN
42. Your answers should include the ideas that:
    a. society bombards us with the message that slimness is necessary for beauty and acceptance. This creates unreasonable expectations.
    b. eating disorders may be a method of avoiding and diverting attention from family conflicts.
    c. brain dysfunction, especially in the hypothalamus (which plays a role in hunger and eating) may predispose a person to develop an eating disorder.
43. learning
44. internalizing
45. Your answers should include the ideas that:
    a. antidepressant medications have had mixed success in the treatment of bulimia and little success in the treatment of anorexia nervosa.
    b. there has been some success using behavior techniques, such as desensitization and cognitive-behavioral therapy.
    c. family therapy, which focuses on clarifying relationships, developing boundaries and improving communication, is often used in conjunction with behavioral therapy in the treatment of anorexia nervosa.
46. enuresis, encopresis
47. a. urine alarm
    b. dry-bed training
    c. medications
48. biofeedback training and parental reinforcement of appropriate toileting

Chapter 4 - Developmental and Learning Disabilities

1. a. 1. lifelong impairment in mental or physical functioning that is first evident prior to adulthood
        2. substantial limitations in daily living skills, such as communication and self-care
        3. the necessity for extended specialized care
    b. infancy and early childhood
2. a. Your answer should include the idea that developmental domains describe general characteristics and skills which are incorporated by children as they develop and are necessary to function adequately.
    b. The typical developmental process and ages at which infants and children are expected to show certain levels of skills is often used as a standard for defining

developmental disability.
    c. 1. motor skills
        2. language / communication skills
        3. cognitive skills
        4. adaptive behaviors
3. 1. h.
    2. i.
    3. g.
    4. f.
    5. c.
    6. a.
    7. d.
    8. e.
    9. b.
4. a significantly subaverage intellectual functioning occurring before the age of eighteen
5. a. 1. how to best distinguish average and subaverage intelligence
        2. whether mental retardation is better defined by cognitive defects or problems in adaptive behavior
    b. Your answer should include the idea that the IQ test score used to distinguish retarded from normal has changed often over the years.
    c. No, specific areas of adaptive functioning are also considered in assessment.
6. 1. moderate
    2. severe
    3. mild
    4. profound
    5. mild
    6. severe
    7. profound
    8. moderate
7. 25 - 50 percent, below
8.

DOWN SYNDROME	
Description of chromosomal abnormality	21st pair of chromosomes fails to separate, resulting in three chromosomes (trisomy)
Description of physical characteristics	eyes are slanted with small folds, body is shorter-than-average and stocky, small hands & short fingers
Description of "aging process"	premature aging -- wrinkled skin and dementia by middle age
Description of typical social characteristics	sociable, stable emotions, good mental health
Common IQ range	IQs typically around 50
Description of typical level of adaptation	Expressive language is most affected, but rote learning & visual-motor skills are relatively well developed so they can learn many life skills with relative ease.

9.

FRAGILE X SYNDROME	
Description of chromosomal abnormality	heritable genetic mutation on X chromosome
Description of physical characteristics	long thin face, broad flat nose, large ears, enlarged testicles in males
Description of typical social characteristics	lack of interest in social relationships, often comorbid with ODD and ADHD
Common IQ range	varies, cognitive effects more severe in males
Description of typical level of adaptation	varies, effects more severe in males

10.

WILLIAMS SYNDROME	
Description of chromosomal abnormality	deleted gene on chromosome 7
Behavioral limitations	vocabulary and hearing abilities far exceed cognitive skills
Description of physical characteristics	elfin appearance -- small turned-up nose, full lips, small chin; heart defect

11.

PHENYLKETONURIA - PKU	
Effect on protein metabolism due to inherited gene mutation	newborn lacks enzyme necessary to convert common amino acid in diet to another amino acid and this results in a toxic buildup which affects the nervous system
Common IQ range if left untreated	about 25 on average
Common IQ range if detected early and treated	in the 90 range
Description of typical behavioral characteristics	moderate to severe retardation, hyperactivity and possibly fearful and bizarre behavior

12. a.   Teratogens are substances that cross the placenta during pregnancy and damage the fetus. Examples are cocaine, tobacco, alcohol and marijuana.
    b.   Your answer should include the ideas that physical effects include small head circumference and facial abnormalities, as well as retarded growth. Behavioral effects include mental retardation, attention problems and learning disabilities.

13.   problems associated with labor and delivery, head injuries, brain tumors, infectious diseases

14.   mild, cultural-familial, have limited intellectual skills or little education

15. a.   examination of prospective parents' family history and blood analysis of chromosomes to predict the chance of child having genetic disorder
    b.   programs focus on young mothers and try to foster good physical and psychological health practices, which in turn may lower environmental risks
    c.   medical testing for early detection, so that further damage can be reduced
    d.   two-generational intervention, including parenting and life skills education for parent and enriched environment for child

16. a.   maximize the child's developmental progress and adaptive behavior skills
    b.   eliminate or reduce disruptive or self-injurious behavior
    c.   help families adjust to the child's disability

17.   Your answer should include the idea that behavior modification programs are based on conditioning principles in which target behaviors are shaped by either reinforcing closer and closer approximations of desired adaptive skills or punishing self-injurious or disruptive behaviors.

18.   Your answer should include the idea that self-instruction attempts to teach children with retardation to monitor their own behavior by following a set of rules which help them stay on task, even in the absence of an instructor.

19. a.   Some children with retardation may suffer from abnormal regulation of endogenous opiates (pain relieving chemicals in the brain). The release of these natural opiates during self-injurious behavior may reinforce the behavior.
    b.   It is believed that self-injurious or other disruptive behaviors may be one of the few ways that the child can interact and communicate with others.

20.   an institution, normalization, all children with mental retardation, self-contained classrooms in regular public schools, increased, mainstreaming

21. a.   1.   severe defects in establishing reciprocal social relationships
         2.   nonexistent or poor language skills
         3.   stereotyped patterns of behavior, activities or interests
    b.   spectrum, all, atypical

22.   Your answers should include the ideas that:
    a.   gross impairment in reciprocal social interaction is a defining feature in autism. Children with autism often seem to look through, rather than look at, other persons.
    b.   spoken language is either absent or minimal in about half of the individuals with autism.
    c.   insistence on sameness is pervasive and often rules the individual's behavior.

23. a.   Persons with autism generally show some degree of mental retardation, while many persons with mental retardation show limited language development.
    b.   Children with retardation usually engage others socially and show reciprocal interaction and use whatever language they possess to communicate with others. Also, while children with retardation show uniformly low scores on intelligence tests, the scores for children with autism vary.

24. a.   Some genetic syndromes like fragile X produce autistic characteristics. The incidence of autism is higher for identical twins than for fraternal twins. The rate of

autism among siblings is higher than that for the general population.

b. Individuals with autism have a higher incidence of physical anomalies, EEG abnormalities and seizures than that of the general population.

c. Structural and functional brain abnormalities have been found using brain imaging techniques. Some studies have found that serotonin levels are higher in the brains of autistic persons.

25. a. Autism is the inability to form attachments.
b. The primary deficit in autism is the inability to imitate.
c. The fundamental deficit is the infant's inability to focus on the mother's face and voice.
d. The focus must be on the individual's inability to infer the mental states of others (theory of mind).
e. The focus should be on the problems associated with executive brain functioning, such as planning, flexible problem-solving and inhibition of off-task behavior in a goal-directed situation.

26. higher, expressive language, greater
27. less, females, 6-18 months
28. Your answer should include the idea that autism and other pervasive developmental disorders are very difficult to treat successfully. Medications, behavior modification and special education have had little success, although certain aspects of these disorders can be improved, especially with behavior modification.
29. Many organizations use their own different definitions which are based on what they emphasize as the cause.
30. Learning disorder is diagnosed when achievement in reading, writing or mathematics is substantially below that expected for the age, schooling and level of intelligence.
31. dyslexia, most, 80 percent, linguistic, phonemes
32. Your answers should include the ideas that:
a. the incidence of reading disabilities is higher-than-average in the children of parents who are poor readers. Rates for identical (monozygotic) twins are higher than for fraternal (dizygotic) twins. Some researchers estimate that genetic factors play a role in about 30 percent to 40 percent of cases.
b. studies show that different areas of the brain are structurally different in those with reading disabilities.
c. poor readers are given less attention in the classroom.
d. parents influence reading readiness, that is the child's expectations for success, motivation and emotional responses to failure.
33. Educational intervention, 5-7, phonic, meaning

Chapter 5 - Stress, Sleep, and Adjustment Disorders

1. stressors
2. a. the nature and timing of the stressors
b. the psychological characteristics and social context of the person
c. the biochemical variables that influence the stress response
3. Your answers should include the ideas that:
a. severe traumatic events such as natural disasters, victimization or sudden loss are surprisingly frequent and can leave lasting psychological scars.
b. many potential stressors occur predictably and regularly as a person moves through his or her live. These include marital difficulties, loss of a loved one, etc.

c. some occupations, especially those that make many demands but allow little control, can be particularly stressful.
d. even common everyday events (arriving late for work or class, losing or breaking something) can be significant stressors.

4. a. Poor social skills or long-term psychological disabilities may increase the chance of unintentionally bringing about stressful events.
b. One stressor often leads to other stress producing situations.
c. Severe stressors may cause physiological changes in brain chemistry, which in turn can contribute to future problems.

5. a. poverty, discrimination in housing and jobs, single parenting and pressure to conform to norms of the majority culture
b. sexual assault, single parenting
c. economic problems, death of loved ones, chronic illness, loss of physical abilities, discrimination brought on by loss of physical attributes emphasized in our culture

6. different, more
7. The accurate statements are:
a. Unexpected stressors take more of a toll on a person than do predictable ones.
b. People usually perceive a stressor as less harmful when they have social support.
c. The perceived negative effects of stressors dramatically increase when people feel helpless or unable to control the situation.
d. A stressor is usually perceived as more harmful when the person knows that it was caused by the intentional or careless behavior of someone else.
e. People who are confident, optimistic and have higher self-esteem tend to be less threatened by stress.

8. 1. a.
2. b.
3. c.
9. a. E
b. A
c. R
d. A
e. R
f. E

10. autonomic, sympathetic, parasympathetic
11. a. Your answer should include the idea that in response to a sudden stressor the hypothalamus produces CRH which signals the pituitary to release ACTH causing the adrenal glands to release adrenal corticosteroids. These stress hormones stimulate the sympathetic nervous system, while inhibiting the parasympathetic system.
b. Your answer should include the idea that the hypothalamus influences the release of the catecholamines epinephrine and norepinephrine.

12. They are special endogenous opioids (naturally produced opiates in the brain) which help regulate cardiovascular activity, relieve pain and facilitate psychological coping with stress.
13. Your answer should include the following: attention to stressor becomes more focused, the rate that people under stress think and perceive the situation is changed and time distortions often occur.
14. 1. d.
2. b.
3. c.
4. h.
5. a.
6. g.

7. f.

8. e.

15. a. Stress hormones, especially corticosteroids affect the immune system by damaging the body and suppressing functioning.

    b. In the short run, it is adaptive because it is necessary to divert needed energy to other bodily functions for quick fight or flight. With prolonged immune suppression, however, the person is susceptible to disease and slowed recovery from illness.

16. coping

17. a. Your answer should include the idea that the goal is to change the stressor itself, or if they can't eliminate it, attempt to change the way that they perceive it through cognitive reappraisal.

    b. Your answer should include the idea that people attempt to reduce the stress by changing their feeling about the stressor, often by using defense mechanisms.

    c. Your answer should include the idea that a powerful method for coping with stress is to seek and use social support. It's important for the person to feel a sense of belonging and that others truly care.

18. a. Social support acts as a buffer that enables people to neutralize the harmful effects of stress.

    b. Social support provides a feeling of belonging that strengthens the person and makes the effects of stress less harmful.

    c. The fact that a person has high levels of social support and low levels of stress may be due to the fact that the person is extremely competent in the first place.

19. a. Anxiety, helplessness, frustration, hostility, sleeplessness and demoralization are the most common effects of stress. Severe stress, however, contributes to several specific mental disorders.

    b. Today, we categorize physical illnesses which are triggered or worsened by stress such as heart disease or ulcers, under the heading Psychological Factors Affecting Medical Condition.

    c. Recent research indicates that stress may play a role in the onset of depression, bipolar disorder and schizophrenia.

    d. The significance of stress for mental disorder is reflected on Axis IV of the DSM-IV.

20. 1. e.

    2. d.

    3. c.

    4. g.

    5. b.

    6. a.

    7. f.

21. four to six, first, immune system replenishment, stage 2 and REM, dreaming

22. a. a rhythmic schedule controlling biological functioning, which repeats approximately every 24 hours

    b. in an area of the hypothalamus called the suprachiasmatic nucleus (SCN)

    c. a hormone produced in the pineal gland when our eyes sense darkness that helps regulate sleep and wakefulness by signaling the hypothalamus and SCN

23. are not, dyssomnias, parasomnias

24.

COMMON DYSSOMNIAS	TYPICAL FEATURES
Primary Insomnia	trouble falling or staying asleep, affecting about 1/3 of U.S. population, especially women
Infant Sleep Disturbance (ISD)	trouble falling asleep, nighttime waking and distress, can precipitate marital discord and child abuse, affects 15-25 percent of infants
Primary Hypersomnia	excessive sleepiness, prolongs episodes of sleep
Narcolepsy	sudden attacks of REM sleep accompanied by cataplexy (muscle paralysis causes body collapse and immobility)
Circadian Rhythm Sleep Disorder	sleep disturbance caused by mismatch between a person's natural circadian rhythm and demands of environment

25.

COMMON PARASOMNIAS	TYPICAL FEATURES
Nightmare Disorder	repeated frightening dreams that interrupt sleep, occur in REM sleep, frightening nightmares common in children under age five
Sleep Terror Disorder	occurs in NREM sleep, person awakens in terror and panic, hard to calm down, no memory of the event next morning, 5 percent of children, 1 percent of adults
Sleepwalking Disorder	occurs in NREM sleep, person leaves bed and moves around or does other simple behaviors, no memory of the event next morning

26. The use of medication is most common, but psychological treatments such as relaxation techniques and sleep hygiene counseling are also used.

27. a stressor, three months, six months, frequently, few

28. Yes. Generally, if a person feels that he or she is handling a stressor adequately, no diagnosis is made. If the person cannot maintain normal functioning or feels enough distress to seek professional help, adjustment disorder is often diagnosed.

29. Adjustment disorders result from stressors of various magnitudes, PTSD is diagnosed only if the stressor(s) were of extreme magnitude. Also, the symptoms of adjustment disorder are more mild and of shorter duration.

30. Answers will vary depending on your personal example.

31. a. Your answer should include the idea that problem-solving therapy helps the person learn to cope with the direct stressor. Effective problem-solving involves defining the problem clearly, identifying possible strategies, evaluating consequences, identifying alternative tactics, choosing and implementing the tactic and assessing effectiveness.

b.   Your answer should include the idea that having the opportunity to express feelings about the stressor (emotional disclosure) is important. It reduces negative thinking patterns and feelings, helps the person think about the situation in a new way and helps the person develop a stable optimistic outlook (dispositional optimism).

c.   Your answer should include the idea that the first step toward enhancing social support is to help the person elicit and accept support from others.

Chapter 6 - Psychological Factors and Health

1.   a.   one-third
      b.   one-third
      c.   one-third
2.   a.   a specialty in psychology, founded in the 1970's and devoted to studying, "psychological influences on how people stay healthy, why they become ill and how they respond when they do get ill."
      b.   1.   understanding how psychological and physiological factors interact to influence illness and health
            2.   identifying risk factors for sickness as well as protective factors for health
            3.   developing and evaluating techniques for promoting healthy behaviors and preventing unhealthy ones
            4.   developing and evaluating psychological interventions that contribute to the effective treatment of illness
3.   The biophysical model holds that physical illness is an outgrowth of biological vulnerability, psychological processes and social conditions.
4.   1.   d.
      2.   c.
      3.   e.
      4.   a.
      5.   b.
5.   a.   Axis III concentrates on general medical conditions that are related to medical disorder.
      b.   The DSM-IV provides special rules for classifying mental disorders caused by drugs and medical conditions.
      c.   It directs clinicians to use multiple diagnoses to classify all the conditions that might apply to a patient.
6.   Your answers should include the ideas that:
      a.   this category is used to describe situations in which psychological factors have contributed to actual physical damage to the body.
      b.   this category describes situations in which a person complains of physical symptoms, but there is no diagnosable physical reason to account for the symptoms.
      c.   this category describes situations in which a person is intentionally faking or exaggerating physical symptoms in order to play the sick role.
      d.   this category describes situations in which a person is intentionally faking or exaggerating physical symptoms for other than psychological gain. This is not a mental disorder.
7.   Your answers should include the ideas that:
      a.   disease can cause psychological changes, such as feelings of depression. Also, behavioral changes including mood swings, can occur when the body's immune system is

called into action.
      b.   disease and psychological conditions may each be influenced by a common, underlying biological process.
      c.   psychological and social influences may exert a direct influence on biological processes, that in turn are implicated in the cause of disease.
      d.   psychological and social influences may indirectly lead to diseases because they are associated with unhealthy behaviors.
8.   strong, heart and circulatory, one-half, stress and personality differences
9.   1.   d.
      2.   g.
      3.   c.
      4.   e.
      5.   b.
      6.   f.
      7.   a.
10.   a.   Your answer should include that Manuck exposed monkeys to threatening stimuli and found that those with the highest response also had significantly more problems with atherosclerosis. In another study, Manuck found that monkeys living in unstable groups developed significantly more arterial plaque than did other monkeys.
      b.   yes
      c.   when the stressor is chronic; when the stressor exceeds the person's perceived ability to cope
11.   Black Americans, men, older people
12.   a.   Type A
      b.   Type B
      c.   Type A
      d.   Type B
      e.   Type A
      f.   Type A
13.   a.   content
      b.   how he or she responds to frustrating incidents occurring during the interview
14.   a.   1.   Your answer should include that the WCGS consisted of an eight and one-half year study of 3,500 men. It found that Type A men were more than twice as likely to have heart attacks than Type B men.
            2.   Your answer should include that the Farmington study of 1,600 men and women found that in an eight year period more than twice as many Type A participants had developed CHD as Type B persons.
      b.   No. The vast majority of Type A's never developed CHD. Also, more recent studies have found that Type A behavior, in general, isn't necessarily a risk factor for CHD.
15.   hostility, especially when it involves cynicism and chronic suspiciousness or distrust of others, as well as anger
16.   overreact physiologically to, more and more, overreact, increase, rapid swings in, weaken
17.   a.   In cancer patients treated with chemotherapy, nausea and vomiting occurring in the twelve hour period preceding drug administration.
      b.   learning (classical conditioning)
      c.   hypnosis, relaxation training with guided imagery and biofeedback

18.

ACQUIRED IMMUNE DEFICIENCY SYNDROME (AIDS)	
What are the specific effects of HIV on the immune system?	HIV destroys the immune system's T cells.
What are the secondary effects of HIV on body function?	The effects include: susceptibility to many types of secondary infections, nervous system damage, malignancies and death.
Why is HIV difficult to control with drug therapy?	HIV can rapidly mutate into new drug resistant strains.
How is HIV transmitted?	Through the exchange of bodily fluids, most notably blood and semen.
How many people are HIV positive in the world today? By the year 2000?	Today, approximately 18 million people are HIV positive. By the year 2000, 30-40 million people will be.
Which two groups have the largest number of AIDS cases in the U.S. today?	homosexual males, intravenous drug users
HIV infections are increasing rapidly in which groups in the U.S.?	low income Black and Hispanic American adolescents and young women

19. a. 1. Most AIDS cases can be prevented by avoiding heavy use of alcohol or drugs before sexual activity, sexual activity with multiple partners or partners with an unknown sexual history, sexual activity without condoms.
        2. The sharing of needles used to inject drugs is a high-risk behavior.
    b. A person's ability to cope with the stress of the disease is directly related to the efficiency of the immune system.
20. orderly, proteins and protein, a tumor, controls cell growth, three
21. a. The incidence of cancer in the United States is mildly linked to ethnicity and gender.
    b. Unhealthy behavioral habits, such as smoking or eating fatty foods, increase the risk of several types of cancer.
    c. Some studies indicate a Type C, cancer prone personality.
22. Your answers should include the ideas that:
    a. people with multiple problems, such as mental illness, tend to drift down to the bottom of the social ladder. This view does not work well, however, when considering physical health.
    b. people with low SES are more often exposed to

environmental hazards such as poor diet and lack of medical care.
    c. that low SES is related to increased rates of negative and potentially harmful emotions, such as depression and hostility.
    d. that people of lower SES face more negative life events, such as poverty and crime, while at the same time they possess fewer resources to adequately deal with these stressors.
    e. that many unhealthy behaviors such as smoking, drug abuse and unhealthy diet, are more common among less educated, lower SES persons. This group is also more resistant to programs designed to modify these behaviors.
23. a. Stress reduction techniques are used such as relaxation training, biofeedback and hypnosis.
    b. Cognitive restructuring is a technique in which patients are taught more adaptive ways to think about problem solving, their illness and their ability to exert control over their lives.
    c. The intervention often takes place in a group setting, which increases social support.
24. a. obesity, cigarette smoking, sodium levels, LDL cholesterol levels, aerobic unfitness, serious stressors
    b. yes, with counseling, yes. Studies show that heart attack reoccurrence dropped significantly when Type A counseling was included as part of the medical treatment.
25. Your answer should include cognitive/behavioral techniques, which often include group training, designed to reduce high-risk behaviors through education, skills training, role playing and group support. Also, clean needle exchange programs and condom distribution are common. Last, but importantly, there are many diverse programs worldwide which are designed to empower women to take better control of their lives and reduce their risk.
26. Your answer should include the idea that cognitive-behavioral stress management (CBSM) programs, which include assertiveness role playing, training in muscle relaxation, cognitive restructuring and basic information about HIV risks and transmission, as well as aerobic group exercise, have been shown to lessen the emotional distress and slow the decline of immune system functioning.
27. a. Your answer should include the idea that educational programs, as well as individual, group and behavioral therapy, have been shown to reduce distress in cancer patients, while also increasing physiological functioning and lessening reoccurrence rates.
    b. At this time, research cannot support this.
28. correct, compliance
29. a. 1. educating patients about the importance of compliance, so that they will take a more active role in maintaining their own health
        2. modifying the treatment plan in order to ease compliance
        3. using behavioral and cognitive-behavioral techniques to increase patient ability to stay in medical compliance
    b. 1. Some examples are postcard reminders, telephone calls, watches with alarms to remind patients to take medication.
        2. These are contracts between patient and physician which spell out and reward compliance behaviors.
        3. Compliance behaviors earn points, which can be exchanged for tangible rewards.
        4. This is often used to reduce avoidance behavior and anticipatory nausea, especially with cancer patients undergoing chemotherapy.
30. a. use of tobacco
    b. abuse of alcohol and illegal drugs

c.   faulty eating habits
d.   infrequent use of seatbelts
e.   failure to obtain and comply with necessary medical treatment
f.   risky sexual practices

31. a.   1.   eating a balanced diet
         2.   getting adequate sleep
         3.   engaging in physical exercise
         4.   using seatbelts
     b.   Changes in lifestyle can be inconvenient and time consuming. Also, positive changes can be gradual and not as immediately reinforcing as unhealthy behaviors.

32. Your answer should include the idea that this model assumes that the most important variables regarding compliance are (1) how the person sees the seriousness of the illness and their susceptibility to it, (2) how effective the treatment is compared to how costly or difficult they perceive it to be, and (3) how motivated they are by internal cues (for example pain) or external factors.

Chapter 7 - Anxiety Disorders

1.   most, the world, one-fourth, twenty-eight
2.   a.   cognitive distress
     b.   physiological arousal
     c.   behavioral disruptions and avoidance
3.   Fear refers to a response to a specific perceived danger, while the term anxiety is usually used to describe a more vague sense of apprehension that something threatening may occur.
4.   a.   It is a less and less frequently used term, usually associated with Freud, which refers to chronic anxiety, unhappiness and guilt which resulted from repressed content.
     b.   no
5.   Anxiety and fear are biologically-based emotions which have adaptative value, but when they go awry, the result may be disfunction.
6.   an irrational, excessive, significantly interferes with everyday life
7.   a.   commonly diagnosed
     b.   women, Black Americans and Hispanics
8.   objects or situations, little or no
9.   a.   In order to meet the DSM-IV criteria for specific phobia, extreme distress occurs whenever the person is or anticipates being exposed to the feared situation.
     b.   In order to meet the DSM-IV criteria for specific phobia, the intensity level of the fear must be intense enough to interfere significantly with the person's life.
10. Your answers should include the ideas that:
     a.   animal phobias are the most common type of specific phobia. They generally develop early in life and most commonly revolve around snakes, mice, spiders, cats and dogs.
     b.   this is another common cluster which usually develops by the early teens. Persons with these phobias often faint and/or avoid medical care.
     c.   this cluster is also relatively common and can include many different stimuli, such as enclosed places. Feared stimuli also often revolve around the natural environment, such as the fear of height or storms.
11. evaluated, embarrassed
12. a.   Common situations include speaking or performing in public, meeting strangers, using public restrooms or dressing rooms and eating or writing in public.

b.   Generalized social phobia involves the fear and avoidance of virtually all public or social situations. This is much more distressing and disruptive than fearing a single particular situation.
13. Your answers should include the ideas that:
     a.   phobic fears rise from unresolved conflicts and repressed sexual urges.
     b.   phobic fears are learned through classical conditioning, while avoidance behaviors are learned through operant conditioning. Observational learning and modeling also influence behavioral development as well as our perceptions of the environment.
     c.   research suggests a genetic influence in the development of phobic disorders, as well as neurotransmitter malfunctioning, resulting in low levels of the inhibitory transmitter GABA and increased stimulation of the amygdala.
     d.   some persons may be biologically "prewired" to overreact to certain types of stimuli.
14. 1.   f.
     2.   d.
     3.   c.
     4.   b.
     5.   a.
     6.   g.
     7.   e.
     8.   h.
15. panic attacks, suddenly, minutes or hours, other attacks will occur
16. a.   Your answer should include the idea that agoraphobia is the most commonly treated phobia by clinicians. It revolves around open spaces and usually involves the fear of leaving home alone, being in public or traveling.
     b.   Agoraphobia often develops from a history of panic attacks. The person anticipates the chance that an attack could occur during a situation which would be especially difficult to deal with, such as being away from home.
     c.   drug and alcohol abuse, depression, increased risk of premature death
17. Your answers should include the ideas that:
     a.   the psychoanalytic view emphasizes unconscious conflict arising from separation anxiety caused by the physical and or emotional absence of the parents.
     b.   panic disorder and agoraphobia tend to run in families, which suggests a genetic component. Perhaps, this is due to biologically caused hypersensitivity to substances or events which are related to panic.
     c.   panic attacks result from misperceptions of bodily sensations or environmental events. These reactions can become learned alarms which create anxious apprehension.
18. a.   Problems reflect a misinterpretation of physical sensations as signs of danger.
     b.   1.   breathing retraining to learn to reduce breathing rate
         2.   interoceptive exposure to somatic cues that trigger attacks
         3.   cognitive restructuring
     c.   yes
     d.   Your answer should include the idea that panic control treatment entails the usual treatment techniques plus educating clients about how panic arises from their tendency to overreact and catastrophise physical sensations.
19. antidepressants and anxiolytics (antianxiety drugs such as the benzodiazepines). Yes, but they can produce problematic side effects.
20. a.   Your answer should include the idea that obsessions are

unwanted, disturbing, often irrational thoughts, feelings or images that people cannot get out of their minds.

b. The obsessions and compulsions seen in OCD are viewed by the person as unpleasurable and uncontrollable.

21. Your answer should include the idea that compulsions are repetitive, nearly irresistible acts that temporarily neutralize obsessions or relieve the anxiety they cause.

22.
a. O
b. C
c. O
d. C

23. Your answer should include the idea that Tourette's disorder is a genetic disorder related to and often comorbid with OCD. It is characterized by the presence of both vocal and motor tics and in about one third of cases, coprolalia (verbal obscenities).

24. Your answers should include the ideas that:
a. researchers are looking into genetic factors for OCD, because there seems to be a general connection between genetic inheritance and predisposition for other anxiety disorders.
b. researchers are looking into low serotonin levels, as well as differences in brain activity in persons with OCD.
c. the cognitive-behavioral view revolves around the assumption that OCD is best understood as a vicious cycle of physiological reactivity and obsessive thinking which increases with stress. The obsessive thoughts increase anxiety levels. Ritualistic behaviors and compulsive responses may reduce the anxiety temporarily, which is reinforcing.

25.
a. Your answer should include the idea that cingulotomy is a rarely used form of psychosurgery successful only in a minority of patients.
b. Your answer should include the idea that clomipramine is a drug that blocks the reuptake of serotonin. It is effective about 50-75 percent of the time.
c. Your answer should include the idea that exposure and response prevention are two effective cognitive-behavioral therapies where the client is exposed to the stimulus that elicits obsessive thoughts, but is kept from performing obsessional rituals.

26. chronically, numerous minor events

27.
a. women
b. persons under age 30
c. young Black males
d. lower socioeconomic status

28.
a. It is difficult to focus on the disorder, because many researchers are unsure if GAD is a separate disorder, or if it is a general characteristic of anxiety and/or depression.
b.
1. Your answer should include the idea that constant worry may be an attempt to maintain tight control over all aspects of one's life.
2. Your answer should include the idea that constant worry may function as a way to actually avoid the emotional or physical feelings of anxiety.

29.
a. Your answer should include the idea that cognitive-behavioral therapy is generally based around cognitive restructuring (identifying and replacing irrational thoughts with less anxiety producing rational beliefs) and relaxation training. These techniques are somewhat effective.
b. Your answer should include the idea that drugs are the most commonly used treatment for GAD, including antidepressants, benzodiazepines and newer nonbenzodiazepines such as buspirone.

30.
a. frequent reexperiencing of the event through intrusive thoughts, flashbacks and repeated nightmares and dreams
b. persistent avoidance of stimuli associated with the trauma and general numbing of emotions

c. increased physiological arousal resulting in increased startle responses or difficulty sleeping

31. acute stress disorder

32.
a. The extent of injury or the victim's perception of potential danger and their inability to control the situation are variables that relate to the development of PTSD symptoms.
b. Risk of developing PTSD is inversely related to the amount of social support that the trauma victim receives after the event.
c. Some studies show that persons are more likely to develop PTSD symptoms if they
1. are overly concerned with bodily aches or pains.
2. have exhibited social maladjustment.
3. are passive, inner-directed and have more aesthetic interests.
4. have been highly sensitive to criticism and are suspicious of others.
d. Some studies suggest that the same genetic factors which predispose persons for panic attacks may also increase the chance of developing PTSD symptoms.

33. Your answers should include the ideas that:
a. a neutral stimulus can be associated with the fear or pain which occurs during a traumatic event. Later, that neutral stimulus can become a conditioned stimulus for anxiety and fear.
b. following a traumatic event, a memory network is set up that interconnects all of the fear stimuli and response elements associated with the trauma.

34. Your answers should include the ideas that:
a. the person is directly exposed to the feared stimuli, whether it be imaginal or in vivo.
b. cognitive therapies often involve the exposure to feared stimuli in the absence of negative consequences. It is assumed that this will alter the memory network. This is often coupled with cognitive processing therapy and cognitive restructuring techniques.
c. no single drug has been found to reduce all of the various PTSD symptoms, however, medications are sometimes used to help manage some of the specific symptoms.

Chapter 8 - Dissociative and Somatoform Disorders

1.
1. c.
2. b.
3. g.
4. d.
5. a.
6. e.
7. f.

2. pathological, common and perfectly normal

3.
a. daydreaming and fantasizing to the point that a person is so absorbed that they lose track of what is going on around them; also, the imaginary playmates and role play of children
b. when it is disturbing to the person and interferes with their ability to function

4. Yes. Your answer should include the idea that speaking in tongues, spirit possession and various trance states are commonly seen throughout the world.

5.

KEY SYMPTOMS	DESCRIPTION OF KEY SYMPTOMS
Amnesia	significant loss of memory, including memory of identity or of a person's past, which is not due to organic causes
Depersonalization	persistent feelings of detachment, including out-of-body experiences and control
Derealization	sense that external world is somehow strange or unreal or has changed in some manner
Identity Confusion	an uncertainty about the nature of a person's own identity, of who he or she is
Identity Alteration	behavioral patterns suggesting that the person has assumed a new identity

6. multiple personality disorder; uncommon; increased; separate; women; childhood trauma, such as extreme abuse

7.
1. b.
2. c.
3. a.
4. d.

8.
a. Your answers should include the ideas that:
   1. DID appears to be a culture bound syndrome usually diagnosed in the United States and Western Europe.
   2. the symptoms of DID include many features which overlap with other disorders.
   3. many of the features of DID can be created through suggestion.
b. Your answer should include the idea that several of the physical and behavioral symptoms commonly seen in DID would be very hard for a person to mimic or fake.

9. sudden loss of memory for personally important information, which often follows a stressor, and is not caused by a medical condition or other mental disorder

10.
1. c.
2. e.
3. a.
4. b.
5. d.

11.
a. Generalized amnesia coupled with traveling to a new location. In some cases, the person in a fugue state becomes confused about their identity and assumes a new one.
b. Most last only a few days, but they can go on for several months.
c. traumatic events or overwhelming everyday stressors
d. In most cases, the person behaves normally.

12.
a. Your answer should include the idea that the central features are distressing depersonalization and derealization which are reported as dreamlike feelings of detachment, where the person feels like he or she and/or the world around him or her is somehow different.
b. Both depersonalization and derealization often accompany other physical and mental disorders as well as drug induced states.

13. Your answers should include the ideas that:
a. some people may become more easily immersed and completely absorbed in daydreaming and internal fantasy. This may make them more prone to dissociative problems.
b. persons who are more open to hypnotic suggestion may be more prone to dissociative problems.
c. it is believed children often use dissociation as a way of dealing with traumatic abuse. This may predispose the person to dissociative problems later in life.

14.
a.
   1. Your answer should include the idea that young children, who are subjected to extreme chronic abuse, are relatively powerless to deal with the situation. They then dissociate in order to cope. Because they are in the process of forming their personalities, the fragmentation becomes part of their identity, and later in adulthood, DID.
   2. Your answer should include the idea that the value of this model is uncertain, because it is often difficult to establish the exact pattern of abuse that took place and many people who were abused as children do not develop DID. Recent research, however, has suggested a possible link between childhood abuse and biological effects on the brain.
b.
   1. Your answer should include the idea that the sociocultural model argues that DID is a role that persons with psychological problems take on, often with the unintended encouragement of therapists.
   2. Your answer should include the idea that although this theory might help to explain some cases of DID, it does not explain all cases of DID.

15.
a. that the individual alters are integrated together into a whole
b.
   1. developing trust between patient and client
   2. working to establish communication and cooperation between the alters, begin to recognize past trauma
   3. strengthening coping mechanisms, work through grief that comes with knowledge of past trauma, begin integration process
   4. client learns to cope with new way of living

16. without formal treatment, triggering stressor

17. This occurs because both problems often accompany other more global disorders such as depression which is treated with medication, psychotherapy or both.

18.
a. NO
b. YES
c. NO
d. YES

19. Somatization is a process by which emotional distress is converted into physical symptoms. This concept is basic to many, but not all, of the somatoform disorders.

20.
a. Factitious disorder describes a category of mental disorder in which a person exaggerates or pretends to have symptoms in order to be seen as sick by others. He or she needs to assume the patient role.
b. No, they differ because the underlying reason for pretending to have symptoms is different. The malingerer is deliberately faking symptoms in order to gain reward (for example, win a law suit) or avoid something (for example, the child pretends to be sick to avoid going to school).
c. With somatoform disorders, the person perceives his or her physical problems to be real. This is not true with the other two disorders.

21. Because symptoms tend to mimic physical medical disorders, this becomes the focus. Also, many patients and physicians view medical illness as more acceptable than mental illness, so

psychological explanations are less likely to be considered.

22. Your answer should include the idea that somatization disorder describes a chronic pattern of many different physical complaints for which no underlying physical explanation can be found, but are serious enough to warrant the desire for medical treatment or interfere with daily functioning,.

23. To diagnose somatization disorder, at least eight different symptoms must have been reported. To diagnose undifferentiated somatoform disorder, six.

24. Your answer should include the idea that hypochondriasis describes a chronic concern that many varied, but common physical sensations, actually indicate the presence of a serious medical illness.

25. The person with somatization disorder has a specific complaint for which they are seeking medical relief. The person with hypochondriasis seeks reassurance that a common physical sensation does not indicate a major medical illness. Also, somatization disorder generally focuses on one physical complaint at a time, while hypochondriasis tends to skip from concern to concern quickly.

26. Your answer should include the idea that in conversion disorder, the person, often after a stressor, experiences problems with motor or sensory abilities (for instance their arm becomes paralyzed or they suddenly go blind). The loss of function suggests a neurological cause , but none exists.

27. a. motor problems
    b. sensory problems
    c. seizurelike symptoms

28. a. a seemingly indifferent and nonchalant attitude toward loss of function, which is often seen in conversion disordered patients
    b. Malingerers tend to display a pattern of behavior opposite that of la belle indifference when discussing their alleged problem.

29. Your answer should include the idea that pain disorder describes a situation where a person's chief clinical complaint is pain, for which psychological factors are thought to be the predominate cause.

30. If the duration of pain disorder is less than six months, it is called acute pain disorder. If the pain lasts six months or longer, it is called chronic pain disorder.

31. Your answer should include the idea that body dysmorphic disorder describes an all consuming preoccupation with one's appearance. The normal looking person sees himself or herself as having a physical imperfection which is believed to be hideously ugly to others.

32. The preoccupation with the imagined imperfection causes tremendous anguish and keeps the person from functioning adequately .

33. Your answers should include the ideas that:
    a. a predisposition to somatoform disorders is conveyed by a combination of biological and psychological vulnerabilities.
    b. the biological and psychological vulnerabilities interact with stressors from the environment which cause physical arousal.
    c. the symptoms of physical arousal are interpreted by the person as signs of physical illness

34. Your answers should include the ideas that:
    a. studies have shown a possible link between patterns of impulsive behavior and the development of somatization disorder.
    b. conversion disorder symptoms generally are on the left side of the body. The left side of the body is controlled by the right hemisphere of the brain, which is also involved with negative emotions. Perhaps this is one of the links between negative emotions and conversion disorder symptoms.

c. the concept of somatosensory amplifiers describes the enhanced perception of normal bodily sensations. Perhaps, this is biologically-based and predispose some people toward hypochondriasis.

d. some people are prone to concentrate on internal sensations and private thoughts. If this tendency is extreme or prolonged, it could predispose people toward certain somatoform disorders.

e. the personality trait of negative affectivity may convey a vulnerability to somatoform disorders because these people tend to worry, be pessimistic, fear uncertainty, feel guilt, tire easily and have poor self-esteem.

f. family attitudes and behaviors about illness help to shape a person's view of illness and could predispose him or her toward somatoform problems. This is especially true in families where illness is a way to gain attention and affection.

g. children with recurrent abdominal pain do not differ from other children, but tend to grow up in families where multiple illnesses are common, mothers describe themselves as sickly and illness is rewarded.

35. Your answer should include the idea that young children who are not able to express themselves verbally may use illness to convey emotional distress, especially those children living in abusive situations.

36. Your answer should include the idea that the role of secondary gain in the development and maintenance of somatoform disorder assumes that the reinforcing qualities of illness are learned as a way to gain attention, avoid stressful responsibilities and express negative feelings.

37.

SOMATOFORM DISORDER	TYPICAL TREATMENT(S)
Somatization Disorder and Hypochondriasis	help patients to better cope with stressors, person works with patient to reduce Dr. shopping and dependence on medical system
Conversion Disorder	hypnosis, behavioral techniques, psychotherapy to help deal with triggering stressor
Body Dysmorphic Disorder	medication, cognitive therapy designed to challenge negative beliefs about appearance, exposure-response therapy
Pain Disorder	combination of behavioral intervention, psychotherapy and medications

Chapter 9 - Mood Disorders and Suicide

1. group of emotional disorders, an even and productive emotional state, affective disorders, depression

2. Mood disorders can interfere with almost all aspects of a person's functioning, including: work, social relationships, enjoyment of life and physical health.

3. There may be a connection, but the specifics are unclear. Perhaps, bursts in creativity cause emotional problems or vice versa. Another possibility is that there may be a common link.

4. a. The depressed mood lasts for much longer, i.e. weeks,

months or even years.

b.   The depression impairs the person's ability to function.

c.   There is a cluster of other physical and behavioral symptoms.

5.   five, twice, are not, at any age

6.   a.   alcohol and other drug abuse, associated legal, financial and interpersonal problems, anxiety and panic attacks, suicide

b.   mixture of anxious and depressive symptoms

7.

BEHAVIORAL AREA		TYPICAL SYMPTOMS
Mood Symptoms (most common)	What is the effect on mood?	dull despair, constant sadness
	How does the person view his or her life?	loss of ability to enjoy activities central to life
Physical Symptoms	What is the effect on appetite?	appetite usually decreases
	What is the effect on energy level and movement?	lack of energy, slow movements
	What is the effect on somatic complaints?	increased complaints about upset stomach or aches and pains
	What is the effect on sleep?	difficulty falling asleep, getting back to sleep
	What is the effect on the immune system?	immune system impaired, increased vulnerability to illness
Cognitive Symptoms	What is the effect on self-esteem?	low self-esteem, guilt, feelings of worthlessness
	Is concentration affected?	yes, difficulty concentrating
	Who does the person blame?	self-blame
	How do they view the future and past?	grim about past, pessimistic about future

8.   a.   psychotic symptoms including delusions and hallucinations

b.   The delusions and/or hallucinations are consistent with the person's depressed thinking.

9.   It is important because family physicians are often the first health care professionals to see the depressed person. This is because the somatic complaints associated with depression often send people to their family doctor first, because the physical symptoms of major depressive disorder can also stem

from other medical conditions.

10. months, three-quarters, five to six, twenties

11. A major depressive disorder is preceded or followed by dysthymic disorder.

12. 1.   d.
     2.   f.
     3.   c.
     4.   e.
     5.   b.
     6.   a.

13. Your answer should include the idea that dysthymic disorder is a chronic ongoing depressive state which is disruptive, though less debilitating to the person's life than major depressive disorder and lasts at least two years.

14. a.   This diagnosis is used when depressive symptoms are quite brief and follow a specific stressor.

b.   This diagnosis is used when depressive symptoms develop from the normal grief reaction. This is not considered a mental disorder, though it can be disabling and the person may seek help.

15. manic-depressive, an extremely elevated, rapidly, within the same day

16. Your answers should include the ideas that:

a.   major depressive disorder is more common in women, while men and women are at equal risk for bipolar disorder.

b.   bipolar disorder usually begins at an earlier age than does major depressive disorder.

c.   bipolar disorder seems to be more frequent among higher socioeconomic status groups than is major depressive disorder.

d.   compared to unipolar depression, bipolar disorder is less often triggered by psychosocial stressors.

e.   bipolar disorder may have a greater genetic basis than major depressive disorder.

17.

	TYPICAL SYMPTOMS
What is the effect on mood?	mood is elevated, expansive or irritable
What is the effect on sleep?	lessened, only a few hours a night
What is the effect on speech?	rapid and pressured, often loud
What is the effect on judgement?	poor, engage in ill-advised, dangerous, promiscuous behaviors
What is the effect on thought processing?	racing thoughts
Is concentration affected?	yes, poor concentration, they are easily distracted
What is the effect on sense of self-esteem?	inflated (grandiosity)

18. Your answer should include the idea that although mania and hyperactivity share problems of excessive behavior, mania also includes additional problems of mood and thinking. Although bipolar disorder may reach psychotic proportions, psychosis always describes an inability to comprehend and perceive events accurately.

19. 1.   c.

2. b.
3. d.
4. a.
5. e.

20. Your answer should include the idea that cyclothymic disorder describes chronic (more than two years) fluctuation between depression and mania that are not severe enough to warrant a diagnosis of bipolar disorder.

21. a. play, bipolar, unipolar, unipolar depression, dysthymia
    b. No. Not everyone who is closely related to a depressed person becomes depressed and some depressed people are the only people in their families to display the disorder. Lastly, genetic models do not explain how genetic endowment leads to depression.

22. a. Low levels of norepinephrine lead to depression and high levels of norepinephrine lead to mania.
    b. Your answer should include the idea that other neurotransmitters including serotonin and dopamine are also involved, that not only the amount, but also the interaction between neurotransmitter may be important and both long and short-term changes in neurotransmitter function may be at work.

23. a. Perhaps low levels of serotonin simply predispose the person to a mood disorder in general and norepinephrine activity determines the specific mood dysfunction.
    b. Perhaps it is a problem with the neurons themselves, rather than the neurotransmitter level.

24. Your answer should include the idea that as a response to stressors, the hypothalamus and pituitary gland send messages to the adrenal glands to release adrenaline and cortisol. Many depressed patients have increased levels of cortisol, which may indicate a problem in the hypothalamic-pituitary-adrenal axis.

25.

THEORY	SUMMARY OF MAIN POINTS
Psychoanalytic Theory (Freud)	Depression is the result of unresolved conflicts involving the loss of a childhood caregiver. This creates dependency and fragile self-esteem.
Attachment Theory (Bowlby)	Children with insecure attachments to adults do not learn to recognize distress and seek support.
Interpersonal Theories	Unsatisfactory relationships in childhood or as adult increase risk of depression due to lack of social support.

26.

THEORY	SUMMARY OF MAIN POINTS
Reinforcement Model (Lewinsohn)	Depression results from environmental situations which decrease positive reinforcement and increase punishment.
Self-control Model (Rehm)	Depressed person's self-evaluation is based on excessively high standards and he or she concentrate on and explain events in terms of failure and negative self-image.

Learned Helplessness	If people feel that they have no control over events, they learn a sense of helplessness and hopelessness.
Cognitive Theory (Beck)	People vulnerable to depression use negative self-schemas and distorted thinking patterns to perceive themselves and world around them.
Self-awareness Theory	Self-focused attention, which produces self-regulation, become over-critical and depressive.

27. a. A diathesis, such as genetic inheritance or problems caused by dysfunctional social relationships, predispose the person to environmental triggers which then combine and result in depression.
    b. a major loss such as death of a loved one, divorce or unemployment, etc.

28. a. focusing attention and activities away from the stressor and onto something else
    b. Distraction may soften the stressor and lessen the severity and length of resulting depression by providing temporary relief as well as increased social support from others.

29. a. endlessly focusing on, thinking about and talking about the stressor or depression
    b. Rumination often enhances the negative effects of the stressor and increases the severity and length of resulting depression.

30. a. a heightened sensitivity to isolation, fear of abandonment and a strong need for love from others
    b. Yes. They are more likely to become distressed over set-backs in their personal relationships.

31. a. They include perfectionism, guilt over failure, self-criticism and a feeling that one is not living up to standards.
    b. Yes. They are more likely to become distressed over work-related failures or loss of status.

32.

CAT.	TRADE NAME	EFFECTS
MAO Inhibitors	Nardil Parnate	increases levels of norepinephrine and serotonin by blocking enzyme that breaks them down
Tricyclics	Tofranil Elavil Norpramin	increase levels of serotonin and norepine-phrine by blocking their reuptake
SSRIs	Prozac Zoloft Paxil	increase levels of serotonin by blocking reuptake
	Wellbutrin	increases levels of dopamine by blocking reuptake

33. a. the most commonly used medication for the treatment of bipolar disorder
    b. Lithium may be toxic and manic-depressive cycles must be watched closely in case a depressive cycle is

beginning.
c.   anticonvulsants such as carbamazepine and valproate
34. a.   Clinicians noticed that psychotic and depressive symptoms were sometimes lessened in patients following spontaneous seizures.
b.   They are administered only to one side of the head, medication to relax muscles and control heart rate and oxygen are given.
c.   ECT is often effective with patients who do not respond to antidepressant medications.
35. Your answer should include the idea that it is an effective treatment for depression with seasonal pattern. It consists of exposing the person to bright light during the early morning hours.
36. Your answers should include the ideas that:
a.   traditional psychodynamic therapy attempted to change the patient's personality structure by exposing and working through various unconscious conflicts. Today, psychodynamic therapy is more directed at the depression itself and is less time consuming.
b.   behavioral therapy tries to alter behavior by reducing depression and increasing positive healthy actions.
c.   cognitive-behavioral therapy revolves around education, behavioral and cognitive techniques designed to change problematic thinking patterns and negative assumptions clients hold about themselves and the world.
d.   the aim of interpersonal therapy is to enhance the patient's support system by working with the patient on life and interpersonal skills.
37. The results of studies vary, so it is still unclear at this time.
38. Medication is used to control the manic symptoms and psychotherapy is employed to help the patient cope with the problems associated with his or her manic behaviors.
39. 15 percent, eight, a previous suicide attempt
40. a.   Women make more suicide attempts, men achieve more completions.
b.   Young persons attempt more suicides. Older persons complete more suicides.
c.   European Americans
d.   depression, alcoholism, schizophrenia
41. It is comparison of the risk of the person's suicidal behavior to the availability of rescue or help in the situation. This is an indication of the actual intent of the person to complete the suicide.
42. a.   increase, 2,000, White, males
b.   1.   While the suicides of older persons tend to be in response to chronic problems, the trigger for adolescent suicide is often a more common acute stressor.
2.   A common precipitating event in teen suicide is hearing about another person's suicide.
3.   Suicide pacts are formed with friends that plan to die together, often for no clearly identifiable reason.
43. There is no consensus at this time.
44. a.   strongly related
b.   1.   b.
2.   d.
3.   a.
4.   c.

Chapter 10 - Schizophrenia

1.   psychosis, hallucinations, delusions, disorganized, crazy or insane
2.   No, they are very different disorders.
3.

PSY. FUNCTION	PATTERN OF DISRUPTION CAUSED BY SCHIZOPHRENIA
Perception	misperceive what is going on around them, hearing and seeing things not there
Attention	trouble maintaining attention
Thought	disorganized and confused
Emotion	blunted or inappropriate
Behavior	often bizarre and outlandish
Social Interaction	often isolated and withdrawn from others

4.   1.   b.
2.   c.
3.   e.
4.   a.
5.   d.
5.   a.   loosening of associations
b.   ambivalence
c.   autism
d.   affective disturbance
6.   no, one symptom, presence of several, month
7.   Your answer should include the idea that positive symptoms describe distortions in normal psychological functions that produce excesses in behavior. Positive symptoms include: hallucinations, delusions, bizarre behavior, confused thinking and disorganized speech.
8.   a.   They are firmly held beliefs which are not shared by other people. The delusional person experiences the world as others do, but forms incorrect interpretations of those experiences.
b.   There are different levels of implausibility and sometimes the beliefs are not held by the clinician's culture, even though they are endorsed by the patient's culture.
9.   1.   a.
2.   d.
3.   e.
4.   g.
5.   f.
6.   b.
7.   c.
10. a.   The process of misattributing internal sensations such as thoughts, daydreams or mental images to external sources.
b.   An illusion is a misinterpretation of an external stimulus, while hallucinations develop from internal events.
c.   1.   auditory hallucinations
2.   tactile hallucinations, visual hallucinations, as well as gustatory (taste) and olfactory (smell) hallucinations
11. delusions and hallucinations, formal thought disorder, speech
12. 1.   c.
2.   d.

3. a.
4. b.
5. e.
13. a. Your answer should include the idea that catatonia describes disordered behavior which can range from immobility to extreme activity and agitated excitement.
    b. inability to function in a focused and patterned manner, includes inappropriate and odd actions
    c. poor hand-eye coordination and clumsiness
14. Your answer should include the idea that negative symptoms involve a lessening, absence or loss of normal functions including: apathy, flat emotions, lack of self-help skills and social withdrawal.
15. Your answers should include the ideas that:
    a. flat affect describes an emotionless state where the person stares straight ahead, with a glazed look, unresponsive to events going on around him or her.
    b. alogia describes slow, delayed or lack of conversational responses.
    c. avolation describes a behavioral state where patients sit for hours on end making no attempt to do anything.
16.

PSYCHOTIC DISORDER	TYPICAL FEATURES	HOW IT DIFFERS FROM SCHIZ.
Brief Psychotic Disorder	sudden onset of positive symptoms following stressor	episode lasts from one day to less than one month, while schiz. requires six months
Schizo-phreniform Disorder	symptoms similar to schizophrenia	lasts more than one, but less than six months, less disruptive
Schizo-affective Disorder	hallucinations or delusions with mood swings	schizophrenia lacks mood swings
Delusional Disorder	nonbizarre delusional beliefs	delusional disorder lacks other schiz. symptoms
Shared Psychotic Disorder	psychotic symptoms induced by another person	causal factor differs from schizophrenia
Substance-Induced Psychotic Disorder	hallucinations and delusions result from ingested substances	causal factor differs from schizophrenia

17. a. about 30
    b. yes
18. a. Hallucinations and delusions are prominent in schizophrenia, but not in autistic disorder.
    b. In schizophrenia, speech is disorganized; in autism, it is severely limited or absent.
19. Your answers should include the ideas that:
    a. the prodromal phase describes a slow gradual descent into schizophrenia.
    b. the active phase usually occurs after a stressor and includes obvious positive symptoms such as

hallucinations and delusions.
    c. the residual phase describes the period where the person has passed through the active phase, but is no longer showing obvious positive symptoms.
20. a. 1, all, higher
    b. all, high
    c. equal for men and women, males, females
21. Because the disorder displays itself in so many different patterns of symptoms, demographic characteristics and impairments, it could easily be a number of different disorders being described by only one name.
22. 1. b.
    2. e.
    3. d.
    4. a.
    5. c.
23. Your answers should include the ideas that:
    a. process schizophrenia describes a pattern of early onset, progressive deterioration (prodromal phase), poor premorbid adjustment and poor prognosis.
    b. reactive schizophrenia describes a pattern of later, sudden onset which often follows a traumatic event, good premorbid adjustment and better prognosis.
    c. Type I schizophrenia describes mostly positive symptoms, good premorbid adjustment, sudden onset and typically responsive to drug treatment.
    d. Type II schizophrenia describes mostly negative symptoms, poor premorbid adjustment, gradual onset and are generally unresponsive to drug treatment.
24.

	SCHIZ. RUNS IN FAMILIES AND IS GENETICALLY TRANSMITTED	GENES ALONE CAN'T ACCOUNT FOR THE DEVELOPMENT OF SCHIZOPHRENIA
Family Aggrega-tion Studies	Studies all show that the closer a person is genetically to schiz., the greater the chance of development.	Very few relatives of those with schizophrenia have the disorder themselves.
Twin Studies	Concordance rates are highest for MZ twins.	Not all MZ twins of schizophrenic parents develop the disorder.
Adoption Studies	Adopted children of schizophrenic mothers have higher rates for the disorder.	Not all children of schizophrenic mothers develop the disorder.

25. a. No single dominant or two recessive genes cause schizophrenia. Different genes act together to influence the development, probability and severity of the disorder.
    b. The diathesis (predisposition) for schizophrenia may be a physical characteristic or personality feature which is acted on by an environmental trigger to bring about symptoms of the disorder.
26. a. It is often found that the twin diagnosed with schizophrenia has decreased brain volume, density or function which is not found in the cotwin.
    b. viral infection early in life, complications during

pregnancy and/or childbirth

27. Your answers should include the ideas that:
    a. the frontal lobes which are involved in planning, decision making and abstract thinking are often found to be decreased in volume and diminished in blood flow in schizophrenics. This may account for various negative symptoms.
    b. irregularities in the temporal lobe and parts of the limbic system which lie underneath have been tied to schizophrenic symptoms, including hallucinations.
    c. the thalamus is a major relay station of the brain, filtering, sorting and transmitting information throughout the entire cortex. Irregularities in the thalamus have been found in schizophrenic patients.

28. a. dopamine
    b. An excess of dopamine is related to schizophrenia.
    c. The excess dopamine hypothesis is too simplistic to explain fully the relationship between schizophrenia and neurotransmitter function.

29. a. HR studies are prospective designs (following participants from an early age to adulthood) which focus on children who are thought to be predisposed to schizophrenia by virtue of having been born to a parent with schizophrenia.
    b. Your answer should include the idea that HR studies suggest that being born to a parent with schizophrenia is a reasonably good indicator of developing serious psychological disorder, including schizophrenia.

30. a. urban, lower
    b. 1. As persons develop the symptoms of schizophrenia, they cannot function adequately and slip down on the socioeconomic ladder.
       2. As urban areas decay, the most able move away, leaving those less able to function, including those with mental disorder such as schizophrenia, behind.
       3. Chronic psychological and social stressors, social disorganization and greater environmental hazards associated with living in poverty, breed new cases of schizophrenia.

31. a. Your answer should include the idea that the researchers once believed that the schizophrenogenic mother, who was domineering, cold, overprotective, rigid and uncomfortable with sex and intimacy, as well as double-bind communication which was comprised of conflicting messages, were both major causal factors in the development of schizophrenia.
    b. no
    c. It caused (and still causes) family members to incorrectly feel that they are to blame for their child's schizophrenic disorder.

32. a. Your answer should include the idea that EE describes emotional exchange between schizophrenic patients and their families. These exchanges include high levels of criticism, hostility and overinvolvement.
    b. EE is not related to the original onset of schizophrenia, but is related to relapses of it.

33. neuroleptics, blocking, dopamine

34. Your answers should include the ideas that:
    a. Parkinsonism describes motor disturbances which are similar to those seen in Parkinson's disease.
    b. acute dystonia describes uncontrollable muscle contractions or spasms of the head, neck, tongue, back and eyes.
    c. acute akathesia describes a condition in which the patient is consistently restless and agitated.
    d. tardive dyskinesia describes a side effect which is associated with long-term use of neuroleptics. TD includes grotesque uncontrollable jerks, tics and twitches

of the face, tongue, trunk or limbs.
    e. neuroleptic malignant syndrome is a potentially fatal disorder which involves extremely high fever, muscle rigidity, irregular heart rate and blood pressure.

35. It is an atypical antipsychotic drug which acts strongly on D4 dopamine receptors and has less serious side effects than traditional neuroleptics.

36. Your answers should include the ideas that:
    a. self-management and social skills training is designed to teach patients skills necessary to conduct themselves successfully in their daily lives.
    b. family therapy focuses on educating the families of schizophrenic patients about the disorder and training family members in effective problem-solving and communication skills.
    c. psychosocial rehabilitation is a set of different interventions designed to prevent unnecessary hospitalizations, reduce impairments of daily functioning, strengthening living skills and modifying environments to make them more supportive.

Chapter 11 - Cognitive Disorders

1. biological damage to the brain, many different cognitive functions, older people

2. a. lesions to specific areas of the brain
   b. lesions to brain tissue which are spread across the brain or at least to several areas of it

3. a. inability to remember events that happened minutes before
   b. loss of ability to understand written language, while still comprehending speech
   c. failure to recognize familiar people or objects
   d. loss of ability to plan simple behaviors
   e. a clouding of consciousness
   f. profound confusion and disorientation
   g. loss of judgement
   h. difficulties perceiving spatial arrangements or coordinating movement

4. Ageism is a form of prejudice against the elderly.

5. It tells us that they are not true.

6. a. Body flexibility, muscular strength and speed, hearing, vision, sensitivity to taste and smell and balance all decline with age.
   b. Drugs become more effective at a lower dose and are also more likely to be toxic.
   c. Studies show that different mental abilities tend to peak and decline at different ages and at different rates. The rate of decline generally becomes steeper with increasing age, but most older persons are just as able to understand and analyze their world as they were in their younger days.
   d. depression; side effects of medication

7. 1. b.
   2. e.
   3. c.
   4. a.
   5. d.
   6. f.
   7. g.

8. delirium and dementia, a general medical condition, a substance, problems with functioning, anterograde amnesia, retrograde amnesia

9. a. In general, cases of amnesia do not last long, so they tend

not to come to the attention of a clinician.

   b.   The problem develops so slowly that it goes unnoticed.

   c.   Sociocultural diversity may affect test results.

10.

DELIRIUM	
Typical course of onset in children	rapid, often coinciding with a high fever
Typical course of onset in elderly	Slowly. A common pattern is that problems increase at night.
Warning signs of impending episode	increased sensitivity to smells or sounds, mild perceptual distortions, problems judging time or concentrating, increased autonomic functioning, sleep-wake cycle reversed
Effects on consciousness	reduces awareness of environment, engage in preservation
Effects on emotion	Emotional changes are common and include depression, apathy, euphoria, anxiety, fear or irritability.
Hallucinations and delusions	Visual hallucinations and paranoid delusions are common.
Effects on memory	memory for recent events commonly impaired, while memory for event which happened long ago, remain intact
Is course rapid or slow?	rapid, corresponding to the medical condition that caused it
Is complete recovery possible?	Complete recovery is common once underlying cause is treated.

11.   factors associated with aging, including abnormal sodium levels, chronic illness, fever or hypothermia, impaired kidney function, changes in living conditions, impaired vision and hearing as well as increased use of prescription drugs

12.   head trauma, postoperative states, drug use, toxins, epilepsy, metabolic disturbances, dehydration and infections

13.   Your answer should include the idea that the major goal of treatment is to identify the underlying causes of the delirium. Associated factors include: support, reorientation, minimize medications when possible, avoid the use of restraints and appreciate and protect the dignity of the patient.

14.   a.   Your answer should include the idea that the major symptoms of dementia include: loss of cognitive functions including memory, thinking, reasoning and concentration to the point that it interferes with daily functioning.

   b.   Dementia has a slower onset, is chronic not acute and is more associated with the elderly.

   c.   Depression comes on more quickly and causes concern for the patient, where dementia comes on more gradually and the person is unaware of the deterioration. Also, depression is often worse in the morning, while dementia worsens as the day goes on. Drugs help depression but worsen dementia. Depression usually improves; dementia does not.

15.   a.   Dementia which is caused by cardiovascular conditions,

such as strokes or arterial diseases which interrupt blood flow to the brain.

   b.   yes, the second most common after Alzheimer's disease

   c.   Although they share many symptoms, vascular dementia differs from Alzheimer's disease in that it comes on much more abruptly and the symptoms develop in various steps, as opposed to the predictable, but gradual deterioration seen in Alzheimer's disease.

16.

MEDICAL CONDITION	DESCRIPTION
Pick's Disease	degenerative disease of unknown cause; frontal lobe atrophy of brain causes dementia; rare, mistaken at times for early onset Alzheimer's disease
Lewy Body Disease	abnormal protein deposits (Lewy bodies) cause degeneration of neurons of cortex & brain stem; hallucinations and motor problems common; rare, mistaken at times for early onset Alzheimer's
Parkinson's Disease	movement disorder which affects over one million Americans; dementia is sometimes seen in the late stages of Parkinson's disease
Huntington's Disease	movement disorder which includes facial grimaces, twitches and chorea; later stages may include personality and emotional changes as well as dementia
Creutzfeldt-Jakob Disease	progressive dementia caused by infectious agent
HIV Infection	dementia is seen in one third of persons with AIDS
Syphilis	sexually transmitted infectious agent; once the most common cause of dementia
Head Trauma	memory impairment and other cognitive and behavioral problems can occur, depending on the severity and location of trauma

17.   one-half, four million, doubles, with early onset, more, with late onset

18.   Your answers should include the ideas that:

   a.   in the early stages of Alzheimer's disease, the primary symptoms are usually increased forgetfulness and the loss of ability to cope with changes in the environment or in routines. Increased apathy, flat emotions and withdrawal are also seen.

   b.   in the middle stages of Alzheimer's disease, the primary symptoms are usually increased problems with language, cognitive understanding and perception.

   c.   in the late stages of Alzheimer's disease, the primary symptoms are usually loss of language, inability to find their way, even in familiar places, or care for themselves.

19.   about 8-12 years

20.   many areas but especially the association cortex of the frontal and parietal lobes, the limbic cortex, hippocampus and amygdala

21.   a.   neurofibrillary tangles which are twisted clumps of

protein fibers found in dying cells
    b.   neuritic plaques which are composed of residue of dead neurons and cellular garbage
22. Although the process is still unclear, it is an abnormal form of a common protein which appears to cause the death of neurons in Alzheimer's disease patients.
23. family history, 50
24.

	ONSET?	EVIDENCE OF LINKAGE
21	early	chromosome 21 linked to the amyloid plaques found in the brains of Alzheimer's disease and Down syndrome patients
1	no information	abnormal chromosome 1 found in families of Alzheimer's disease patients, normal in families without
14	early	abnormal chromosome 14 found in families of Alzheimer's disease patients, normal in families without
19	late	chromosome 19 produces the proteins ApoE-2 which may protect against Alzheimer's disease and ApoE-4 which appears to increase risk

25.
    a.   Repeated blows to the head, such as in boxing, have been linked to Alzheimer's disease, but it is now believed that as little as a single concussion may increase risk.
    b.   Heart attacks greatly increase the risk of Alzheimer's disease, especially in women.
    c.   The neurotoxins aluminum and mercury are found in high levels in Alzheimer's disease patients. The relationship is still unclear.
    d.   The brains of persons with Alzheimer's disease have dramatically reduced levels of ACh.
    e.   Alzheimer's disease is found significantly more often in persons lacking formal education.
26. Because clinicians do not know enough about the causes of the disease or the biological mechanisms leading to cell death to develop effective interventions.
27.
    1.   b.
    2.   c.
    3.   a.
    4.   g.
    5.   e.
    6.   f.
    7.   d.
28. Your answers should include the ideas that:
    a.   caregivers need to respond to the patient's immediate emotional, psychological and physical needs.
    b.   caregivers need to respond to the patient's continuing need for emotional and physical closeness.
    c.   caregivers need to recognize that they, themselves, need special help.

Chapter 12 - Personality Disorders

1. personality, personality trait, II, maladaptive
2.
    a.   The personality disorders are ego-syntonic, that is, seen as natural and normal by the person displaying them.
    b.   Personality disorders are very difficult to treat.
    c.   Personality disorders are often more distressing to others than to the person displaying them.
    d.   Personality disorders are often comorbid with Axis I disorders.
3.
    a.   usually by adolescence or young adulthood
    b.   between 10 and 13 percent
    c.   men
4.
    a.   Yes, in fact, it is quite common.
    b.   1.   The Axis I disorder and the personality disorder may simply coexist at the same time, aggravating each other.
           2.   One of the disorders may predispose the person to the other.
           3.   The symptoms of Axis I and Axis II disorders often overlap, causing a duel diagnosis for a single problem.
5.
    a.   Not only do the symptoms of Axis I disorders often overlap with personality disorders, but the symptoms of the different personality disorders also often overlap.
    b.   An accurate social history is necessary for the diagnosis of personality disorders, but this is often difficult to obtain.
    c.   It is especially difficult to apply the DSM categorical approach to personality disorders.
6.
    1.   c.
    2.   a.
    3.   e.
    4.   d.
    5.   b.
7. Your answer should include the idea that the Interpersonal Circumplex is based on the theories of interpersonal psychology and assumes that personality structure can be described as different combinations formed from the basic interpersonal dimensions of dominance-submission and love-hate.
8. Your answer should include the idea that paranoid personality disorder involves long-standing traits of suspiciousness and mistrust. These people are irritable and hostile, often misinterpreting innocent actions or remarks as threats or insults directed at them. Their suspicious view of the world is often reinforced by their own self-fulling behaviors.
9. between 0.5 and 2.5 percent
10. Your answer should include the idea that schizoid personality disorder involves an indifference to social relationships and needs as well as emotional flatness. These persons prefer solitary activities and usually have few, if any friends, which is due to their lack of social skills and the common feelings of pleasure or emotional pain that sometimes go along with social relationships.
11. probably less than 1 percent
12. Your answer should include the idea that schizotypal personality disorder implies behaviors, thinking, speech and belief patterns which, though nonpsychotic, are perceived by others as odd, strange or weird. Whereas the schizoid personality disordered person shuns people for lack of interest, the schizotypal often leads an isolated life because he (and others) feel uncomfortable when together. Schizotypal personality disorder may be genetically linked to schizophrenia and mood disorders.
13. between 2 and 4 percent
14. Your answer should include the idea that the main features of

histrionic personality disorder are attention-getting behaviors which often include seductiveness, exaggerated displays of emotion and demands for reassurance and praise. At first, others may see the histrionic as creative or fun loving, but their self-centered and demanding exhibitions soon drive others away.

15. between 2 and 4 percent

16. Your answer should include the idea that the behaviors of narcissistic personality disordered persons are driven by their overinflated sense of self-importance which gives them, they believe, an inherent right to special privileges and entitlements. Their preoccupation with self results in little concern or empathy for others and destroys social relationships.

17. probably less than 1 percent

18. Your answer should include the idea that the essential qualities of borderline personality disorder are impulsivity and instability in several areas of functioning, including mood, behavior, self-image and interpersonal relationships.

19. a.   about 2 percent
    b.   women

20. moral insanity, psychopathy, sociopathy

21. Your answer should include the idea that antisocial personality disorder describes a pattern of behavior which, because of a lack of moral and ethical development, results in a predatory attitude and actions toward others. A master manipulator, the antisocial personality disordered person is impulsive, unreliable, insincere, disregards the truth, lacks remorse, does not learn from experience and is incapable of feeling genuine emotion, including love for others.

22. Antisocial personality disorder is preceded prior to age 15 by conduct disorder. (See chapter 3)

23. a.   between 3 and 4 percent
    b.   men

24. Your answer should include the idea that the lives of persons with avoidant personality disorder are impeded by their consistent feelings of inadequacy and ineptitude, especially in social situations. They are so afraid of being embarrassed, criticized or ridiculed by others, that they avoid social situations whenever possible. When interacting with others, they are inhibited, timid and overly cautious.

25. about 1 percent

26. Your answer should include the idea that persons with dependent personality disorder are so lacking in self-confidence, they cling to others for reassurance and information on how to live their lives. They are submissive and will make excessive self-sacrifices for the smallest sign of affection.

27. between 2 and 7 percent

28. Your answer should include the idea that the lives of obsessive-compulsive personality disordered persons are hampered by rigid preoccupation with rules, details and minute organization and planning. Every aspect of their lives (and, if they had their way, the lives of those around them) are governed by their inflexible demand for what they consider to be the "right way" to do things. Because of their preoccupation with often unimportant details, these people often are ineffective and indecisive in their actual performance.

29. between 2 and 6 percent

30. Obsessive-compulsive personality disorder describes a chronic lifestyle, as opposed to the specific obsessions and compulsive actions of OCD.

31. a.   genetic influence
    b.   nonshared environment
    c.   shared environment

32. a.   somewhat supports or mixed results
    b.   somewhat supports or mixed results
    c.   somewhat supports or mixed results
    d.   strongly supports

e.   somewhat supports or mixed results
f.   somewhat supports or mixed results
g.   somewhat supports or mixed results
h.   does not support
i.   does not support
j.   somewhat supports or mixed results

33. a.   Your answer should include the idea that traditional psychodynamic theory argued that personality (character) arose from fixations which occurred during the psychosexual stages of development.
    b.   no

34. Your answer should include the idea that object relations theory believes that the nature and quality of early attachments between infants and caretakers will determine how the person expects others to respond to and interrelate with them when they become adults. If these expectations become rigid and extreme, personality disorders can result.

35. Your answer should include the idea that interpersonal learning theorists believe that most personality traits involve interpersonal themes and are both shaped and solidified as a result of interpersonal learning experiences. Personality disorders result when an individual learns to rely too heavily on extreme and maladaptive behaviors toward others.

36. a.   1.   the minimization of pain and the maximization of pleasure
          2.   adapting to environmental demands through passive accommodation or active modification
          3.   advancing the self and caring for others
    b.   As a result of genetic influences, psychodynamics and learning histories, some people develop deficiencies, imbalances or conflicts in one or more of these polarities. The result is personality disorder.

37. a.   Your answer should include the idea that a few studies have found a relationship between organic brain problems and borderline personality disorder. Also, many of the significant symptoms of borderline personality disorder involve mood and biological factors which are known to play a role in the affective disorders.
    b.   The psychoanalytic theorists believe that the construction of self-identity, which is an important aspect in borderline personality disorder and occurs during the first two years of life, can be damaged by the child's aggressive impulses or problematic parenting styles.
    c.   Although the validity of this research is questioned by some, studies suggest that many persons with borderline personality disorder come from abusive backgrounds or have suffered other early trauma.

38. a.   Antisocial personality disorder seems to be related to an underdeveloped cerebral cortex. This may help explain problems with impulsive behavior.
    b.   Persons with antisocial personality disorder tend to have unusually low levels of anxiety and physiological arousal.
    c.   Persons with antisocial personality disorder are probably predisposed biologically to have difficulty learning fear responses.

39. a.   history of parental criminality
    b.   chronic parental uninvolvement, erratic discipline, physical abuse, poor supervision of children
    c.   early loss of parent
    d.   history of social and health handicaps in the family
    e.   exposure to deviant peers

40. most difficult, long-standing, are not, narcissistic

41. Your answer should include the idea that DBT is based on the belief that borderline personality disorder arises when children with emotionally unstable temperament are raised in environments where emotions are tightly controlled, ignored, punished or trivialized. The therapy first tries to help clients

develop basic skills to control their erratic behavior. Then, the problematic experiences are confronted and resolved.

42. a.   no
   b.   Persons with antisocial personality disorder are seldom motivated to change and lack the ability to trust or develop rapport with the therapist.

Chapter 13 - Substance-Related Disorders

1.   substances which affect thinking, emotions and behavior
2.   Billions of dollars are spent manufacturing, advertising and selling drugs like alcohol or nicotine, while at the same time, billions of dollars are spent treating diseases, punishing crime, making up for absenteeism, etc., which are caused by drug use.
3.   a.   increase in criminal activities
   b.   negative prenatal effects on infants
   c.   deaths directly linked to drugs
4.   a.   1.   The level of use is hazardous to one's health.
         2.   The level of use leads to significant impairment in work or family life.
         3.   The level of use produces personal distress.
         4.   The level of use leads to legal problems.
   b.   adverse consequences
5.   a.   desire (craving) for the drug
   b.   increased time procuring and using drugs, reduced time for school, work, family, etc.
   c.   continue to consume drug, even when the user knows that it is causing problems
6.   a.   Also known as addiction, this occurs when physical changes are brought on by excessive and frequent use of a substance.
   b.   1.   tolerance
         2.   withdrawal syndrome
7.   a.   1.   substance use
         2.   substance induced
   b.   abusing several substances at the same time
8.   drug use resulting in recurrent negative social and personal consequences; examples: can't go to school because of a hangover, arrested for drunk driving
9.   continued drug use resulting in negative consequences and indicators of psychological or physiological dependence; examples: stealing money to buy drugs, withdrawal symptoms
10.   Since the 1980's individual alcohol consumption, as well as the number of persons who report that they drink heavily, has decreased slightly. The number of alcohol related deaths has also declined. This is probably due, in part, to a change in social attitudes brought on by increased exposure to information about problems associated with alcohol.
11.   The statement is not true. Even though some problems associated with alcohol have declined slightly, alcohol continues to be a leading cause of mortality, illness and violence in America.
12.   a.   one-third
   b.   one-third
   c.   one-third
13.   stomach (small amount absorbed) - small intestine (most absorbed) - blood stream - other organs (including liver, where it is oxidized)
14.   a.   It will increase.
   b.   1.   Food in the stomach limits the amount of alcohol transported throughout the blood stream to the brain.

2.   Women metabolize alcohol less efficiently than men.
3.   Individuals of Asian descent metabolize alcohol more rapidly than most Caucasians.

15.   1.   b.
     2.   e.
     3.   a.
     4.   d.
     5.   c.
16.   a.   excitatory neurotransmitter; inhibits; diminishes brain cell activity (depressant effect)
   b.   inhibitory neurotransmitter, enhances activity; diminishes brain cell activity (depressant effect)
17.   a.   increases; increases; increases
   b.   Alcohol increases dopamine and serotonin levels in "reward centers" of the brain. Alcohol increases release of endogenous opiates which are similar to opiate drugs which produce euphoria and reduce pain.
18.

BAC	BEHAVIORAL EFFECTS
- .05	relaxation, mild loss of inhibitions
.05 - .08	slurred speech, mild coordination problems
.10 +	noticeable coordination problems; mood, drowsiness, perceptual problem, attention
.25 +	loss of consciousness, death

19.   a.   The sedating effect of alcohol wears off before the agitating effects. This causes a "rebound" of agitation after drinking.
   b.   As tolerance develops due to long-term use, other behavioral effects and personality changes worsen. Example: hostility, aggression, brooding
   c.   Problem-solving skills, especially those involving ability to concentrate and flexibility in thinking, diminish.
20.   a.   circle: males
   b.   circle: young adults
   c.   circle: White European American men who drink
   d.   circle: African American women who drink
   e.   circle: Hispanic American males; underline: Asian Americans (both genders)
21.   a.   1.   prealcoholic: occasional social drinking; relaxation
         2.   prodromal: heavier (often secret) drinking, crucial loss of control when drinking, binges, blackouts, health and social life deteriorates
         3.   chronic: whole life revolves around drinking, malnutrition, physical tolerance, withdrawal symptoms
   b.   1.   Not all alcoholics fit into the different phases.
         2.   The model doesn't fit many female alcoholics.
22.   a.   Type I: late onset, prone to anxiety, binge drinking, unlikely to behave antisocially when drinking, health problems
   b.   Type II: begins in adolescence, little anxiety, antisocial when drinking, fewer medical problems
23.   1.   b.
     2.   c.
     3.   a.
     4.   d.
24.   A single factor theory won't work, because there are many different patterns of drinking and impairment.
25.   a.   The risk of abuse is seven times greater among the first-degree relatives of alcoholics than first-degree relatives of nonproblem drinkers.

b. There is a higher concordance rate among identical twins than for fraternal twins for consumption and susceptibility to effects of alcohol.

c. Adoption studies find that adopted-away children born to alcoholic parents are more likely to develop problem drinking in adulthood than adopted-away children born to nonalcoholic parents. (strongest)

d. Some studies suggest that the D2 receptor may be the genetic marker for alcohol vulnerability.

26. a. Sons of alcoholic fathers have higher than normal beta waves and show less EEG change after drinking. This many show that they are less aware of the effects of alcohol.

b. Alcoholics show less MAO activity than nonalcoholics. Low serotonin levels are related to alcohol craving in animals.

c. Men with a family history of alcoholism show greater increase in heart rate after drinking. This may indicate that they have an increased sensitivity to the stimulating properties of alcohol.

27. a. This hypothesis states that the reduction of tension, anxiety, anger and depression which occurs when drinking alcohol is negatively reinforcing. Laboratory studies support this hypothesis, but studies outside the laboratory have been inconclusive.

b. Many social learning theorists believe that drinking is determined by the reinforcement that an individual expects to obtain. This view has strong research support.

c. Alcoholics tend to rely most on "external" cues to guide their drinking behaviors, while nonproblem drinkers rely on both external and internal cues.

d. Certain personality characteristics seem to correlate with increased chance of problem drinking. These characteristics include antisocial, sensation-seeking, novelty-seeking and undersocialized-aggressive personality traits.

28. a. Parenting style and drinking behavior of parents affects later drinking behaviors of the children.

b. Peer pressure and social acceptance are commonly regarded as important factors in the development of drinking behavior, but research in this area is lacking.

29. 1. c.
    2. b.
    3. a.
    4. b.
    5. a.
    6. a. b

30. 1. a.
    2. b.
    3. d.
    4. c.
    5. b.
    6. d.
    7. a.

31. Because of the tremendous diversity of individual characteristics and treatment programs, the greatest success occurs when therapeutic techniques are matched with the drinker's demographics, drinking style, personality characteristics, motivation and awareness for change.

32. inhibit, sleep, anxiety

33.

	BARBITURATES	BENZODIAZEPINES
Medical Uses	treating anxiety and insomnia	treating auditory and panic disorders, muscle spasms

Effects	relaxation, mild euphoria, impaired motor & cognitive function, depressed blood pressure, depressed respiration	relaxation, euphoria
Health Risks	coma, death	toxicity & overdose when combined with other depressants

34. Your answers should include the ideas that:
    a. depressant use in adolescents is often recreational and done in social settings.
    b. the pattern of depressant abuse for middle-aged or older middle class persons often begins with a prescription for anxiety, insomnia, pain.
    c. the pattern of depressant abuse for the elderly often begins with a prescription for sleep problems. Older persons are more susceptible to the intoxicating effects of the drug and often suffer from memory, cognition and motor problems.

35. physical withdrawal symptoms complicate detoxification; abstinence syndrome complicates relapse prevention.

36. excitatory, increasing, dopamine

37.

	AMPHETAMINES	COCAINE
Medical Uses	asthma, ADD, obesity, congestion	none
Effects	alertness, focused attention, aggressiveness, delirium	rapid stimulation, euphoria
Health Risks	cardiovascular problems, withdrawal, dysphoria	psychological dependence, respiratory and heart failure, death

	CAFFEINE	NICOTINE
Medical Uses	cold remedies, diet pills	none
Effects	mild stimulation, positive mood, nervousness, agitation, anxiety	none discussed
Health Risks	caffeine intoxication, heart disease	cardiovascular & respiratory disease

38. 1. d.
    2. b.
    3. a.
    4. c.
    5. e.
    6. f.

39. narcotics, endogenous

40. Your answer should include the idea that both endogenous

(natural) opiates and exogenous opiates (for example, morphine) influence pain sensitivity and positive mood. When exogenous opiates are frequently ingested, endogenous opiate production is slowed. If the intake of exogenous opiates is stopped, low levels of both will result and both mood and pain sensitivity will be affected.

41.

	OPIATES
Medical Uses	pain reduction
Effects	dulled senses and attention, dream-like euphoria, depression, coma
Health Risks	respiratory failure, intense withdrawal symptoms, death

42. a. Your answer should include the ideas that methadone maintenance therapy may help reduce illicit opiate use, criminal activity and the transmission of infectious diseases. It is also believed that addicts stay in treatment longer on these programs.
   b. Your answer should include the idea that addicts remain dependent and it is argued these programs may actually increase inappropriate drug use.
   c. more

43.

	CANNABIS	HALLUCINOGENS
Medical Uses	anorexia, glaucoma, nausea	none
Effects	mild euphoria, mild perceptual distortions	variable mood, perceptual distortions, depersonalization, paranoid thinking, synesthesia
Health Risks	variable mood, perceptual distortions, depersonalization, paranoid thinking, synesthesia	flashbacks, panic attacks (LSD), fatal overdose (PCP)

44. 1. a.
    2. b.
    3. c.
    4. d.

Chapter 14 - Sexual and Gender Identity Disorders

1. 1. g.
   2. e.
   3. b.
   4. a.
   5. d.
   6. c.
   7. f.
2. They are independent of each other.

3. Alfred Kinsey, representative of, National Health and Social Life Survey
4. a. yes
   b. men
   c. reliving a prior sexually exciting experience or imagining sexual activity with a current romantic partner or with another partner
5. a. Your answer should include the idea that the X and Y chromosomes determine biological sex. Females inherit two X chromosomes, one from the mother and one from the father. Males inherit an X from the mother and a Y from the father.
   b. Your answer should include the idea that during the first 8-12 weeks of development, male and female sexual physiology is exactly the same. At that point, the presence of a Y will determine male characteristics. If no Y is present, female characteristics result.
   c. Your answer should include the idea that androgens (male) and estrogens (female) kick in to produce a variety of primary and secondary sexual characteristics.
6. a. It is an inherited disorder in which the adrenal glands masculinize the external genitalia of females.
   b. A genetic defect on the Y chromosome which causes males to be born with external female genitalia.
7. a. homosexuality listed as a mental disorder
   b. The DSM states that homosexuality itself is not a disorder, but lists sexual orientation disturbance to describe disturbances stemming from homosexual orientation.
   c. name changed to ego-dystonic homosexuality
   d. all references to homosexuality as a mental disorder deleted
8. No, studies have revealed no significant differences in the prevalence of mental disorders or the overall quality of psychological functioning between homosexuals and heterosexuals.
9. most, over 60, 10 percent, high
10. Your answers should include the ideas that:
    a. the results of twin studies have varied and the picture is not yet clear.
    b. early findings from recent research suggest that there may be a particular gene on the X chromosome which relates to homosexual orientation.
    c. recent studies have found differences in the brain structure of homosexuals as compared to the brain structure for heterosexuals in three different areas.
    d. some studies have found that females exposed before birth to abnormal levels of both androgens and estrogens are more likely than comparison groups to become homosexual or bisexual.
    e. a series of studies have shown that male homosexuals tended to be later-born children and come from families with an overrepresentation of male siblings.
11. a. No. Support has been found for biological contributions to homosexuality, but no well controlled study has been able to confirm a clear role for a psychological factor.
    b. no
12. a. persistent cross-gender identification
    b. profound discomfort or even disgust with his or her biological sex and sexual organs
13. a. transsexual
    b. A hermaphrodite is a person who has both male and female sexual organs.
14. a. Boys. Because gender-atypical behavior in little girls is less likely to be condemned by peers and adults.
    b. Children. It is thought that many children outgrow the disorder.

15.

TIME PERIOD	COMMON CHARACTERISTICS / TYPICAL BEHAVIORS
Infancy	gender-disordered boys described as beautiful or feminine babies
Ages 2-3	preference for cross-gender activities and toys, fantasy play at cross-gender roles, prefer to play with opposite sex
Kindergarten	rejection and teasing from other children begins
School Aged	overt cross-gender behaviors suppressed by negative feedback from parents and peers

16. No, and even when they do persist, the overt atypical gender behaviors are less overt.

17. a. individuals who are homosexual or asexual
    b. heterosexual (almost exclusively males)

18. No clear link has been established between genetic factors or brain structure and gender identity disorders.

19. Some researchers have singled out parental indifference as a causal factor in gender identity disorders, but this has not been clearly proven.

20. Your answer should include the idea that psychological treatments for gender identity disorders focus on behavior therapy for the child, including modeling and reinforcing gender appropriate behaviors, parent training, which involves coaching parents about how to reshape their children's behavior, or both.

21. Your answer should include the idea that female-to-male surgery involves breast removal and in some cases an attempt is made to create a fully functioning penis, although this is difficult. Male-to-female surgery involves removal of the penis and the creation of a vagina, hormone therapy and electrolysis for hair removal.

22. a. desire to have sex, often triggered by thoughts and fantasies about sexual activities or partner
    b. increased heart rate and respiration, swelling of penis or clitoris, lubrication of vagina, flushing, breast enlargement, erection of nipples
    c. ejaculation of semen, contractions of the labia minora, vagina and uterus
    d. disengorgement of blood in sexual organs, sense of well-being

23. They were researchers who, beginning in the late 1950's, conducted landmark, detailed laboratory studies of the physiological aspects of the human sexual response and sexual dysfunctions.

24. a. Your answer should include the idea that anything that can negatively impact on neurological or vascular function can disrupt sexual response, including chronic illness, emotional disorders, medications and the normal effects of aging.
    b. Your answer should include the idea that our culture, religious beliefs, family traditions and prior sexual experiences can have a dramatic impact on sexual responsiveness.
    c. Your answer should include the idea that the amount of emotional closeness or distance between partners is an important factor in sexual responsiveness.

25.

HYPOACTIVE SEXUAL DESIRE DISORDER		
Typical Features	infrequent interest in or motivation for sexual activity which causes distress or relationship problems	
Prevalence	between 15 and 40 percent of adults in the United States	
Possible Biological Causes	Men	low testosterone levels
	Women	inconclusive (low estrogen level not a cause)
Possible Psychological Causes	Early Childhood	abuse, perhaps a failure to develop an adequate sense of independence
	Other	depression, negative expectations, unpleasant past relationships, unresolved conflicts about relationship

26. Sexual aversion disorder is similar to HSDD, but more extreme. The person not only lacks desire, but fears or is disgusted by the idea of sexual contact.

27.

SEXUAL AROUSAL DISORDERS		
	FEMALE SEXUAL AROUSAL DISORDER	MALE ERECTILE DISORDER
Typical Features	persistent problems attaining and maintaining lubrication and genital swelling which causes distress	failure to attain or maintain an erection adequate for sexual activity
Prevalence	no information	52 percent over age 40 at some point in their lives
Possible Biological Causes	various (if so, not diagnosed as FSAD)	various (if so, not diagnosed as MED)
Possible Psycho. Causes	childhood abuse	abuse, anxiety, distraction, negative expectations

28.

ORGASMIC DISORDERS			
	Female Orgasmic Disorder	Male Orgasmic Disorder	Premature Ejaculation
Typical Features	inability to reach or extremely delayed orgasm	inability to reach or extremely delayed orgasm	ejaculation before or immediately after penetration which causes distress or interpersonal conflict
Prevalence	difficult to ascertain, perhaps 10 percent	4-10 percent	33 percent
Possible Biological Causes	muscle tone, hormonal, alcohol use	various (although there is little research)	hyper-sensitivity (both bio. and psycho.)
Possible Psychological Causes	lowered sexual desire & arousal	lack of arousal & conflict	learned response, inability to monitor excitement

29.

SEXUAL PAIN DISORDERS		
	DYSPAREUNIA	VAGINISMUS
Typical Features	recurring problems with pain before, during or after sexual intercourse (both men and women)	involuntary muscle spasms of vagina which makes penetration impossible
Prevalence	unknown, of those seeking treatment 5% of women, 1% of men report as primary problem	varies culturally, 5-42% of women seen in American sex clinics
Possible Biological Causes	men - urinary tract infection, certain chronic or sexually transmitted diseases women - various infections, endometriosis	unknown, sometimes occurs with dyspareunia, so it may be related to those factors
Possible Psychological Causes	negative feelings or sexual trauma	classically conditioned avoidance, harsh demanding behavior by partner

30. Your answer should include the idea that Masters and Johnson believed that most problems were due to inadequate knowledge about sexual functioning coupled with performance anxiety. They proposed intensive therapy, which was done daily, for two weeks. First, an exhaustive history was taken, followed by presenting information about sexual functioning, the specific problem and sexual and marital communication. Next, the couple was encouraged to practice sensate focus, a process of relating through physical means which very gradually leads to intercourse.

31. a.   more difficult
    b.   1.   In the cognitive-behavioral approach, the couple is taught to fantasize about sex, investigate how their problems with desire may have developed, uncover and expel irrational thoughts or fears about sex and develop new behaviors.
        2.   the development and alteration of sexual scripts
        3.   medication
        4.   gonadal hormone therapy

32.

	SPECIFIC TREATMENT TECHNIQUES
Female Sexual Arousal Disorder	no specific treatments other than the use of vaginal lubricants
Male Erectile Disorder	various methods, often focusing on anxiety reduction (sensate focus), information to dispel myths about performance and erectile failure, relaxation techniques and communication improvement
Female Orgasmic Disorder	direct training in masturbation coupled with techniques for anxiety reduction and information on sexual response and relationship problems
Premature Ejaculation	squeeze technique, stop-and-start technique, anxiety reduction, medication
Sexual Pain Disorders	use of lubricants, various cognitive-behavioral techniques such as relaxation, sensate focus, fantasy, and for vaginismus, vaginal insertion exercises

33.   repetitive patterns of sexual behavior in which arousal and/or orgasm depends on fantasies or actions involving atypical or socially inappropriate stimuli

34.   1.   g.
    2.   e.
    3.   h.
    4.   c.
    5.   a.
    6.   b.
    7.   d.
    8.   f.

35.   a.   Because rape is a crime of violence, not sex.
    b.   Your answers should include the ideas that:
        1.   one type is the person with a history of sexual aggression and the other antisocial conduct. Often, they were sexually abused as children.
        2.   one type holds callous distortions about women that allow them to justify sexual aggression by believing that the woman wants to be raped and enjoys it. This is common in date rape.
        3.   one type experiences high levels of sexual arousal

from depictions and fantasies of rape; they confuse aggression with sex.

4. the last type experience episodes of depression or hostility, they loose control and become aggressive to women.

36. no

37. Your answers should include the ideas that:
   a. some theories emphasize the importance of sexual stressors in childhood, which interrupt or distort early sexual learning experiences.
   b. classical conditioning may play a role, by associating normal sexual arousal with inappropriate stimuli.
   c. learning may, in some instances, account for paraphilias because sex and aggression are often linked in the popular media and social value sysrem.

38. One of the first techniques used in the United States, which is still in use today, aversion therapy attempts to extinguish the behavior by associating it with unpleasant or painful events. This is often coupled with attempts to replace the problematic stimuli with more appropriate stimuli.

39. Commonly used, this treatment package involves initial establishment of rapport with the client. Next, behavior modification, using masturbatory reconditioning and covert sensitization, is used. Relapsed prevention and the associated emotional defects that contribute to paraphilias are also addressed.

Chapter 15 - Biological Treatment of Mental Disorders

1. drilling of holes into the skull to allow the cause of the mental illness (usually believed to be evil spirits) to escape, most common during prehistoric times through the middle ages, but seen in some cultures even today

2.
   1. c.
   2. e.
   3. f.
   4. b.
   5. d.
   6. a.

3. Because the surgeon was unsure of exactly what areas of the brain were being lesioned, considerable tissue was often destroyed. This caused many side effects including epileptic seizures, impulsiveness, incontinence, lack of planning, poor judgement, lack of motivation and self-care, extreme lethargy and impaired thinking and memory.

4. Using computer-guided imaging techniques, surgeons can now place instruments precisely where they are needed during surgery.

5. Cingulotomy is done by inserting electrodes into a portion of the cerebral cortex in order to lesion an area of the limbic system, which is involved in emotional experience. This surgery can be beneficial in intractable cases of depression and anxiety disorders, especially very severe cases of OCD. Possible side effects can include personality changes and as many as 12 percent of patients commit suicide.

6. SST is similar to cingulotomy, except that a different area of the brain, a region at the base of the frontal lobes, is lesioned.

7. persons with mental disorders involving strong emotion, such as severe depression, bipolar disorder and extremely disruptive anxiety disorders (especially serious cases of OCD) that do not respond to drugs or other treatment

8. a. Psychosurgery is usually performed as a last resort on patients who have not responded to other precise treatment.
   b. It is difficult to compare outcomes of psychosurgery, because diagnostic practices and criteria for success differ.
   c. Psychosurgery outcome studies report treating many types of disorders. It is difficult to tell if overall success rates are affected by the particular mix of clients included in a particular study.
   d. Success rates of psychosurgery cannot be compared with a placebo control.

9. Your answer should include the idea that Sakel believed that the coma caused by insulin overdose was an effective treatment for drug addiction, schizophrenia and other disorders. No.

10. Your answer should include the idea that Meduna believed that seizure disorders and psychosis could not exist simultaneously in the same person, so he induced seizures with metrazol in hopes of finding a cure for psychosis. No.

11. a. Your answer should include the idea that Cerletti and Bini used a very high voltage of electricity to induce grand mal epileptic seizures in patients.
   b. Today, electrodes are placed only on one side of the brain, electrical impulses are of shorter duration and of less voltage, a general anesthetic and muscle relaxant is used to lessen body spasms, oxygen is administered and the patient's brain functions are closely monitored.
   c. Injures and death are rare. headaches, a few hours of confusion and memory loss for up to six months and in a few cases, indefinitely

12. severe mood disorders, yes

13. a. The convulsions associated with ECT correct the imbalance or dysregulations in endocrine and neurotransmitter systems.
   b. An undiscovered substance which regulates mood in the same way that insulin regulates sugar metabolism is stimulated by the repeated convulsions.

14. psychotropic, psychopharmacology, only 27, increasing, grown, up to 90

15. a. Drug treatment is often effective.
   b. Drug treatment is believed by some to be more cost effective than other treatment plans.
   c. Amid controversy, pharmaceutical companies have gained control of many managed care systems and, it is argued, emphasize drug treatments over other techniques.

16. Your answers should include the ideas that:
   a. the drug enhances neural activity because it is chemically similar enough to a natural neurotransmitter to mimic its effects, thereby stimulating neurons to fire. These drugs are called agonists.
   b. the drug (called an antagonist) reduces neural activity because it is chemically similar enough to a natural neurotransmitter to take up space in the receptor site, without stimulating the neuron to fire. This blocks natural neurotransmitters from attaching to the site and stimulating the neuron.
   c. the drug prolongs the availability of neurotransmitters in the synapse by blocking their reuptake.
   d. the drug increases the availability of neurotransmitters by interfering with the natural process that breaks them down.

17. Drugs effect whole categories of neurons in the brain, which can have an impact on many different functions of the body.

18.

DRUG CLASS	MODE OF ACTION	POSSIBLE SIDE EFFECTS
MAO Inhibitors	increase levels of norepinephrine and serotonin by blocking enzyme that breaks them down	elimination of REM sleep, elevation of blood pressure when coupled with diet of foods containing tyramine
Tricyclics	increase levels of serotonin and norepinephrine by blocking their reuptake	sleepiness, dry mouth, constipation, insomnia, blurred vision, decreased sex drive, dizziness, nausea
SSRIs	increase levels of serotonin by blocking reuptake	nervousness, insomnia, joint pain, sweating, weight loss, sexual dysfunction
Heterocyclic Anti-depressant	increase levels of dopamine by blocking reuptake	less effect on sleep and sexual functioning than SSRIs

19. a. 1. A natural effect of aging is that smaller dosages of psychoactive drugs have more impact, so it is easy to overdose.
    2. Well controlled studies have failed to show that antidepressant drugs are helpful to depressed children, even though half experience negative side effects.
  b. Yes.
20. a. lithium carbonate
  b. 1. Lithium may alter secondary messengers in the neuron itself, thereby reducing the availability of dopamine and norepinephrine.
     2. Lithium may stabilize electrolyte balance in the neurons, thereby stabilizing the neuron's reactions to various neurotransmitters and making them less likely to fire.
  c. Yes.
  d. It must be taken, even when the person is symptom free, in order to prevent further episodes.

21.

DRUG CLASS	MODE OF ACTION	POSSIBLE SIDE EFFECTS
Benzo-diazepines	facilitate the post-synaptic binding of GABA, an inhibitory agent, thereby reducing nerve transmission	drowsiness, fatigue, impaired movement, clouded thinking, physical dependency, dangerous interaction with alcohol

Anxiolytics	affects the receptors for serotonin and dopamine	no serious side effects, dependency problems or interaction with alcohol

22. MAO inhibitors, TCAs and SSRIs have been effectively used to treat anxiety disorders, especially panic disorder, agoraphobia and OCD.

23.

DRUG CLASS	MODE OF ACTION	POSSIBLE SIDE EFFECTS
Typical Neuro-leptics (Pheno-thiazines)	dopamine antagonist	Parkinsonism, acute dystonia, tardive dyskinesia, neuroleptic malignant syndrome
Atypical Neuro-leptics (Clozapine)	antagonist with strong impact on the D4 dopamine receptor but less on the D2 receptor, also affects other neurotransmitters	dry mouth, excessive salivation, agranulocytosis -- which is a potentially fatal blood disease

24. a. It increases the effects of norepinephrine and dopamine by increasing release and blocking reuptake.
  b. mimics dopamine
25. reduced food intake, insomnia, abdominal pain, headache, nervous habits and tics, increased heart rate and blood pressure
26. Your answer should include the idea that some critics argue that children may believe that they need medication in order to think, learn and control their own behavior. There is a chance of possible abuse of the drug, use may continue into adulthood and the focus turns to medication and away from education and skills training.
27. Your answers should include the ideas that:
  a. some ethnic groups (Chinese patients in China and African Americans) metabolize TCAs faster and need lower dosages for the same effect than do Caucasians in the United States.
  b. Asians metabolize benzodiazepines more slowly than do Caucasians.
  c. Asians need a lower effective dose than African Americans or European Americans.
28. Your answer should include the idea that lower doses of benzodiazepines and neuroleptics are needed to produce therapeutic responses in females compared with males and females show greater side effects.

Chapter 16 - Psychotherapy

1. a. special training and experience treating people
    b. the ability to show empathy for the client
    c. the capacity for warmly supporting clients
2. No.
3. Yes. Persons from lower socioeconomic groups tend to seek psychotherapy less often and terminate therapy earlier than persons in higher socioeconomic statuses.
4. Clients from different cultural backgrounds have different values and beliefs, which can have a dramatic impact on their ability to participate and succeed in therapy.
5. a.. African Americans
    b. Hispanic Americans and Asian Americans
6. a. 5.
    b. 3.
    c. 4.
    d. 1.
    e. 2.
7. a. Clients treated by nonprofessional counselors do about as well as persons treated by professional therapists.
    b. Novice therapists do about as well as experienced therapists.
8. a. Your answer should include the idea that the most crucial component is the relationship between the client and the therapist.
    b. They can develop an initial therapeutic contract, seek to maintain conditions which will facilitate the continued growth of the therapeutic relationship and act in a professional manner.
9. a. psychoanalytic/psychodynamic
    b. phenomenological/experiential
    c. interpersonal
    d. behavioral
    e. cognitive-behavioral
10. a. They combine the assumptions and procedures from two or more theoretical points of view.
    b. In descending order: psychodynamic, cognitive, behavioral and phenomenological / experiential.
11. unconscious, years, insight, emotionally working through
12. 1. a.
    2. d.
    3. f.
    4. h.
    5. b.
    6. e.
    7. g.
    8. c.
13.

VARIATIONS OF PSYCHOANALYSIS	
THERAPY	MAJOR GOALS / TECHNIQUES
Psycho-analytically Oriented Psychotherapy	They use basic Freudian techniques, but in a more flexible and active manner. For example, there is no couch, there are fewer sessions and there is a more conversational atmosphere.
Ego Analysis	They disagreed with Freud's emphasis on unconscious sexual and aggressive motivation and focused on ego and the person's ability to develop positive adaptive behaviors.
Adler's Individual Psychology	Focus on deep-seated, mistaken beliefs about one's self, which is the cause of disordered behavior. It used dream analysis and direct advice to help adjust thoughts and behavior in order to help client build new lifestyle.
Object Relations and Self Therapy	They believe that the relationships developed between infant and caregivers during the first three years of life forms personality and guides expectations for child as an adult. Therapy is designed to provide gratification missed in infancy.

14. Your answer should include the idea that Sullivan thought mental disorders were caused by the client's inability to develop or maintain positive and healthy interpersonal relationships. The goal of therapy, then, should be to counteract the person's use of ploys and extreme behaviors when dealing with others, by offering feedback and information on how to be more open, honest, flexible and positive with others.
15. Your answer should include the idea that Weissman and Klerman's version of interpersonal therapy, which is used in the treatment of depression, focused on four specific interpersonal problems: 1) prolonged grieving over the loss of a loved one, 2) social role conflicts, 3) difficult transitions and 4) lack of interpersonal skills.
16. a. Phenomenologists believe that the therapist must learn to see and understand the world through the eyes of the client.
    b. P/E therapists have a positive view of human beings and believe that people are not driven by instinct. They place tremendous importance on the concept of free will.
    c. P/E therapists believe that the most important factor in successful therapy is the honest and open relationship between the therapist and the client.
    d. It is important, P/E therapists believe, that patient and therapist are regarded as equals if treatment is to be successful.
    e. P/E therapy emphasizes the experience and exploration of painful or confusing emotions as important to the therapeutic process.
17. The client is asked to imagine that a person, who is associated with conflict in the client's life, is sitting in a chair. The client is then instructed to talk to the imagined person and tell them honestly and frankly how he or she feels. It is hoped that this will help the client increase awareness of unresolved conflicts and emotions.
18. a. Conditions of worth are judgements imposed by others which distort an individual's feeling and actions and hamper personal growth and well being.
    b. a supportive and nonjudgmental relationship
    c. 1. unconditional positive regard
        2. empathetic understanding
        3. all of the therapist's actions and feelings must be genuine and congruent
19. Your answer should include the idea that Gestalt therapy is based on the idea that there are gaps or distortions in people's awareness of their genuine feelings, which cause behavioral problems. Therapy is designed to help the client become aware of the feelings or needs that he or she have disowned and recognize that these feelings and needs are a genuine part of his or herself. To do this, the person must actually reexperience old problematic emotions and feelings.
20. It has broadened its focus to reflect the latest research in

perception, cognition and biological bases for behavior.

21.

BEHAVIORALLY-BASED THERAPY		DESCRIPTION OF MAJOR FOCUS / ELEMENTS
Systematic Desensitization		Used to treat phobias and other anxiety problems, uses relaxation during gradual exposure to hierarchy of anxiety-arousing stimuli.
Exposure Treatments		direct exposure to frightening stimuli until it disappears
Assertiveness Training		training people to appropriately express feelings and emotions through education and practice
Model-ing	Modeling	observations of others engaging in feared behaviors
	Coping Modeling	observations of others first experiencing anxiety, then successfully overcoming it, as the observed person engages in feared behaviors
Contingency Management		presentation or withdrawal of reinforcers or aversive stimuli after engaging in desired behavior
Contingency Contracting	Contingency Contracting	contingency management program with addition of formal agreement between client and therapist
	Token Economy	secondary reinforcers used to alter behavior
Biofeedback		mechanical measurement of biological changes provides feedback necessary to learn to control those behavioral changes
Aversion Therapy		controversial treatment, uses presentation of unpleasant or painful stimuli in hopes of decreasing unwanted behaviors

22. Traditional behavioral therapy focuses on changing overt problematic behaviors, while cognitive-behavioral therapy focuses on that, as well as the maladaptive beliefs and thoughts which so often accompany these behaviors.

23. Beck believes that the negative and distorted beliefs that people hold about the world and themselves are a major factor in many mental disorders, especially depression. It is necessary, therefore, to correct these distorted thinking patterns and replace them with more appropriate and healthy thinking strategies.

24. Ellis believes that anxiety, depression and other problems are brought on by irrational, extreme and self-defeating beliefs. Upsetting emotions may not be the result of an external event, as much as the irrational interpretations of how the person believes that he or she handled the event. The therapist's job is to challenge the irrational beliefs of the client, in order for them to change.

25. randomly, control, experimental, factorial designs

26. a. Nonspecific factors, such as expectations for improvement, the opportunity to talk with an understanding person, the chance to express emotions in a safe environment and receiving encouragement to change, may affect the outcome of the study.

   b. 1. It is virtually impossible to create a psychotherapy placebo which is inert from every theoretical perspective.

      2. The factors that different therapies share, such as creating expectations for improvement and change, may be more powerful in creating change than the specific procedures which differentiate one therapeutic technique from another.

      3. ethical objections

27. the same client, different times, baseline, intervention, ABAB

28. a. Research which is conducted with only one subject.

   b. 1. It allows clinicians to evaluate the treatment of rare disorders.

      2. It encourages practicing therapists to conduct research on their own.

      3. It allows for research to be done at the time that the therapeutic technique is actually employed.

      4. It is less expensive and does not require large numbers of clients or therapists.

29. 1. c.
    2. b.
    3. a.

30. a. single-subject designs

   b. combine resources, clients and talents of many therapy researchers into a large cooperative outcome study being conducted simultaneously at several sites

   c. do psychotherapy research in the laboratory (called analogue research)

   d. Researchers can place a higher premium on external, rather than internal validity by using large surveys, such as the Consumer Reports Survey.

31. No. Research which is specifically designed to maximize one form of validity, must often preclude high degrees of other types of experimental validity.

32. Meta-analysis is a statistical technique which combines the results of several studies into an overall average or estimate. Meta-analysis can help provide needed quantitative information on the effectiveness of psychotherapy, which is an impossible task when so many different qualitatively oriented researchers are using so many different standards and methods to do their research.

33. a. The average person receiving psychotherapy is better off at the end of it than 80 percent of the persons who did not receive therapy.

   b. Deterioration following psychotherapy is infrequent.

   c. The nature of the therapist's professional training is not strongly related to success.

   d. The length of treatment is not strongly related to success.

   e. The specific type of therapy used is not strongly related to success.

Chapter 17 - Alternatives to Individual Therapy

1. 1. d.
    2. c.
    3. a.
    4. e.
    5. b.
2. Alternative therapies seek to change how other people contribute to or are affected by disturbed behavior.
3. a. The high cost of some forms of psychotherapy may be too expensive for many people.
    b. Many people are reluctant to seek psychotherapy because of cultural values or perceived stigma.
    c. There are not enough health care professionals available to provide individual psychotherapy to all who need it.
4. It does not address the social aspects of the disorder, such as social conditions and environmental stressors.
5. If all the focus is on what is wrong with the person, that individual's competencies are overlooked and prevention is impossible.
6. a. Your answer should include the idea that group therapy is designed to allow several unrelated people to discuss their problems with one another under the guidance and leadership of a group therapist.
    b. World War II
    c. Every major theoretical approach is offered in a group format.
    d. Yes.
7. The group format gives clients the opportunity to talk to each other and observe each other's progress as treatment proceeds.
8. a. Sharing new information and insights with other members of the group is helpful.
    b. Group feedback is more powerful, especially when there is agreement among members of the group.
    c. Group members develop positive outcome expectancies when they interact with each other and observe how others change.
    d. Group members learn that they are not the only ones who have problems in general or their kind of problem in particular.
    e. Group members experience helping others.
    f. Dealing with other group members enhances interpersonal skills.
    g. Interactions taking place within the group may allow some members to explore lingering problems caused by maladaptive family interaction.
    h. If group cohesiveness is high, a warm, loving, safe and accepting environment is created for members.
9. six to twelve, homogeneous, heterogeneous, twice, increasing, less
10. a. No.
    b. Effective group leaders must be able to accurately monitor the therapy process, communicate clearly with clients and convey warm support for all of them.
11. a. Yes, especially when group members clearly understand how the group will be run and what is expected of them.
    b. When the group is cohesive, it provides accurate feedback for its members and encourages interpersonal learning and supportive interactions.
    c. There is little evidence that individual psychotherapy is any more effective than similar treatments in a group format.
12. a. Your answer should include the idea that marital (couples) therapy is the psychological treatment of problems in marriages and other intimate relationships.

b. the relationship
c. It is when both members of the relationship see the same therapist in the same sessions.
13. a. The couple engages in the process of rewarding wanted target behaviors which they believe will aid the relationship, while not reinforcing unwanted problematic actions.
    b. Cognitive-behavioral therapists focus on the ways a couple thinks about their relationship and attempts to modify the attributions the couple make about each other.
    c. Emotionally-focused couples therapy tries to help partners feel more comfortable expressing and accepting each other's emotional needs.
    d. Insight-oriented couples therapy focuses more on exploring unconscious conflicts in the relationship.
    e. Employed by almost all therapists, communications training teaches a couple to interact more openly and honestly in order to be able to solve problems together.
14. a. True.
    b. False. Even when improvements are made, as many as half of treated relationships remain distressed.
    c. True.
    d. False. As with most forms of marital therapy, marital enrichment programs have not demonstrated that they can produce lasting changes in long-term relationships.
    e. True.
15. Your answer should include the idea that family therapy is psychological treatment aimed at changing patterns of family interaction to correct family disturbances.
16. a. circular causality (events are interrelated and mutually dependent) In families, no one member is the cause of another's problems. Instead, the behavior of each family member depends to some extent on each of the others.
    b. ecology (systems can be understood not as a collection of parts, but as an integrated whole) In families, a change in the behavior of one member will affect all of the other members.
    c. subjectivity (all of our perceptions of events are filtered through individual experiences) Each member of the family has his or her perception of family events.
17. It is the one member with the most easily identifiable problems. This person is usually the focus at the beginning of family therapy and can often be the vehicle by which aid is made available to others in the family group.
18. In many disturbed families, the main communication patterns involve threats and other coercive messages.
19. a. Teaching family members alternative noncoercive ways to communicate their needs, firm and consistent disciplinary practices, clear communication, behavioral-exchange principles and the development of reasonable expectations.
    b. The focus is on reframing the problem as a breakdown in the system, not as an issue of an individual member.
    c. The therapist asks clients to purposely perform, even exaggerate, problematic behaviors. This may teach the person that he or she is in control of the behavior.
20. a. Yes.
    b. behavioral and structural family therapies
21. Your answer should include the idea that a self-help group is one that meets regularly, without a professionally trained leader, to address members' psychological problems.
22. a. Members usually have a well-defined problem or set of experiences.
    b. Self-help group meetings focus on exchanging information, providing feelings of togetherness and belonging and discussing mutual problems.
    c. Most SHGs charge low or no fees. Their goal is to provide mutual aid, not to make a profit.

d. Most SHGs are member-governed and rely on group members as the primary care givers.

23. 1. a.
    2. c.
    3. d.
    4. b.
    5. e.

24. a. Because the goals of most self-help groups are hard to precisely define.

    b. moderate

25. a. One problem was deinstitutionalization, which was the removal of thousands of mental patients from institutional settings. It was a problem, because there was no place for them to go.

    b. Mental health centers were built, but they could not offer the type of intensive interventions needed to treat the chronic and often psychotic patients who were released from the hospitals.

26. a. Your answer should include the idea that psychosocial rehabilitation teaches patients who display schizophrenia, major mood disorders and other severe disorders how to better cope with the effects of the disorder and how to prevent or lessen the crisis that often threatens their ability to function in society.

    b. 1. The National Alliance for the Mentally Ill
       2. self-help groups
       3. community-oriented mental health professionals

27. a. It involves the empowerment of powerless and dependent people, by teaching formerly hospitalized mental patients basic skills needed to live successfully and independently in the community.

    b. 1. to help a patient understand his or her disorder
       2. to help a patient identify and learn skills needed for community living
       3. case management, to offer assistance in employment, housing, nutrition, finances, transportation, etc.
       4. promote efforts to maintain a coalition among mental health professionals, family members and patients

28. Studies show that psychosocial rehabilitation programs can teach patients life and self-care skills, but performance does decline somewhat when the patient is out in the community. Relapse rates and other indicators of problems are lower for those patients who have gone through comprehensive psychosocial rehabilitation programs. Research findings on long-term effects are mixed.

29. a. Community psychologists believe that behavior must be explained as an interaction between individuals and their environment.

    b. Community psychologists believe that intervention should take place in the settings where the client lives, works or goes to school.

    c. Community psychologists make use of action research, which involves actual changes in the normal operation of social institutions.

    d. Community psychologists put a tremendous emphasis on prevention.

30. 1. c.
    2. a.
    3. b.

31. a. help parents and children form strong and healthy attachments

    b. teach children and adolescents effective cognitive and interpersonal skills, such as problem solving techniques, which will aid them in their development

    c. analyze environments which have a profound effect on development, such as families, schools, neighborhoods

and the criminal justice system, and then change them to make them more supportive

d. reduce environmental stressors and/or help people cope more effectively with the major stressors they must endure

e. promote empowerment by helping those who lack the confidence and the ability to take control of their own lives to develop those characteristics

32.

COMMUNITY PSYCHOLOGISTS HAVE LEARNED THAT:	THEREFORE:
some especially damaging risk factors have widespread effects on human development. (see table 17.3)	these risk factors must receive the highest priority in prevention planning and programing.
most mental disorders are caused by a host of social, economic and psychological risk factors.	to be most effective, prevention programs should be multifaceted and address all of the major risks to the kinds of disorders being targeted.
risk factors tend to have cumulative effects; the longer they occur in people's lives the more serious are their consequences.	because of the domino effect, prevention programs should target risk factors early, before their impact spreads.
certain risk factors are particularly dangerous during specific developmental stages.	to be most effective, programs must be designed to address the right risk factor at the right time in the client's life.
to be most effective, prevention programs need to take into account the cultural norms and values of the people they aim to help.	interventions should be designed to capitalize as much as possible on people's natural strengths, existing resources and cultural traditions, rather than expecting the client to fit into the program.
prevention-centered research is a beneficial tool in the development of new programs.	the development of preventative interventions should be guided by risk factor theories that have been rigorously tested by research conducted in the natural environments where targeted disorders occur.
primary prevention efforts introduce a special set of dilemmas and problems.	prevention scientists must often deal with unintended consequences, ethical questions and difficulties initiating programs and duplicating results of demonstration projects.

Chapter 18 - Legal and Ethical Issues in Mental Disorders

1. It effects society in many ways, including the burden of care from relatives, absenteeism and loss of productivity at work and school as well as direct and indirect costs involved in care.

2. the consideration of the potentially positive and negative therapeutic effects of legal rulings

3. a. Your answer should include the idea that civil commitment was the legal order which made it possible to commit people displaying serious mental disturbances to institutions without their consent. It was commonly used in the 1950's and 1960's.

    b. It was based on the tradition of *parens patriae* ("the country as parent"), which holds that certain types of weakness or impairments can render people incapable of deciding what is best for them. It is the responsibility of the state, much like a parent, to take over and do what is best for a patient.

4. Factors included are the social upheaval of the 1960's, the civil-liberties movement and the strong bias against psychiatry, which was due to its lack of success up to that point.

5. a. the person is mentally ill

    b. the person poses an imminent risk of danger to self or others

    c. treatment is available

    d. hospitalization is the least restrictive alternative for this treatment

6. Your answer should include the idea that deinstitutionalization was a governmental policy of the 1960's which led to the removal of thousands of mental patients from institutional settings.

7. a. It created a revolving door problem of numerous readmissions and short stays in inpatient settings.

    b. Even though the number of inpatients in mental hospitals decreased, admission rates in other types of inpatient services increased.

    c. Many thousands of deinstitutionalized patients became homeless and/or wards of the criminal justice system, because there was no place for them to go which offered needed treatment and support.

8. a. one million, one-third, one-half

    b. impaired judgement, the inability to comply with treatment, inadequate shelter and nutrition, physical illness, unemployment, social rejection and victimization

9. Your answers should include the following ideas:

    a. assertive outreach orientation and integrated case management-- Case workers would actively seek out and provide clients with immediate aid, as well as helping them obtain more permanent support.

    b. safe havens--Temporary protected shelter and basic needs would be provided until more permanent accommodations for the homeless can be found.

    c. integrated system of care and support services--This system would provide various support services including economic support, health care, psychosocial rehabilitation, mental health and substance abuse treatment, education and vocational services.

10. A significant percentage of the homeless mentally ill come into contact with the criminal justice system either because of their disturbed behavior or the unwillingness of the community to accept them. They are often arrested instead of hospitalized. At times this occurs because it is easier for the police to take the person to jail than to commit them to a hospital. Sometimes the hospital will not or cannot admit the person for treatment.

11. In some states involuntary commitment is allowed, if it is believed that a nonviolent person is unable to care for himself and will deteriorate further if not incarcerated.. The "thank-you theory" is based on the idea that individual rights should not be placed above the alleviation of suffering.

12. 1. a.
    2. b.
    3. c.

13. a. Medical patients, after being given information about the possible advantages and disadvantages of a given medical treatment, must give informed consent before that treatment is administered.

    b. no

14. a. No, in some states mental patients can be ordered to comply with any treatment that a professional deems necessary.

    b. no

15. a. This is not an accurate statement. Only about 10 percent of patients refuse treatment and even fewer refuse medication for very long. Some increase in violence may occur, but not to the level expressed in this statement.

    b. This is true, because of the increased time for the clinician, judicial and court costs, waiting periods and review panel objections.

16.

QUESTION	RESPONSE	PRECEDENCE
A group of concerned neighbors comes before the city council demanding that a law be passed which will block the construction of a halfway house for recently discharged mental patients in their neighborhood. Can they do that?	No. Federal laws prohibit housing discrimination against people with mental disorders. (The Supreme Court has also ruled that cities cannot pass laws requiring special permits for homes for mentally retarded patients.)	Fair Housing Amendments Act of 1988 American with Disabilities Act of 1990 Cleburne Living Center v. City of Cleburne Texas
An inmate on death row, who displays the symptoms of paranoid schizophrenia, is judged legally insane. Can he be executed?	No. The Supreme Court has ruled that it is unconstitutional to execute insane people.	Ford v. Wainwright
In many states mentally ill patients have the right to refuse treatment, but do they have the right to be treated and not merely confined?	Yes. Several courts have held that patients have a right to receive more from a mental hospital than just confinement.	Rouse v. Cameron

Can a nonviolent person who can live successfully in the community and has family support be involuntarily confined in a mental institution?	No. The Supreme Court has ruled that simply the need to treat a mental disorder is not enough to justify involuntary commitment.	O'Connor v. Donaldson Foucha v. Louisiana
A mental patient who is not dangerous is put in restraints and food is withheld because she did not make her bed. Although this is obviously unethical, is it illegal?	Yes. The Supreme Court has ruled that an involuntarily committed mental patient has the constitutional right to: (1) adequate food, shelter and clothing, (2) adequate medical care, (3) a safe environment, (4) freedom from restraint unless necessary for protection and (5) training required to ensure rights.	Youngberg v. Romeo (Other individual state laws can and have set higher standards.)

17. 1. b.
     2. d.
     3. a.
     4. c.
18. a. if the therapist believes that the client needs to be involuntarily committed to a hospital
     b. if a client raises the issue of his or her mental condition in a court proceeding and the therapist is called upon to testify
     c. if the client has undergone a court-ordered psychological evaluation
     d. if the therapist learns that the client is abusing other people
     e. if a client tells a therapist of his or her intent to harm another person
19. a. Your answer should include the idea that the Tarasoff decision set a precedent that therapists in California are required to take steps to protect potential victims from clients whom the therapist believes, or should believe, are dangerous.
     b. They believed that without the promise of confidentiality, patients would withhold information important to the therapeutic process or possibly avoid seeking help altogether.
     c. It made therapists more alert to potentially dangerous behavior by their clients. Also, the feared negative impact on the therapist-client relationship has not been as great as predicted.
20. a. A professional relationship had to exist between the client/plaintiff and the therapist.
     b. The therapist was negligent in treating the client.

Negligence means that a reasonable standard of care was not met.
     c. The client/plaintiff suffered harm.
     d. The harm suffered by the client/plaintiff was caused by the therapist's negligence.
21. a. 5 to 8 percent
     b. 1. It has harmful effects on the client.
         2. The therapist is putting his or her needs before those of the client.
         3. The therapist engaging in sexual conduct with a client is not likely to be objective in making judgements about the proper care of that client.
         4. Persons in therapy are often in the midst of psychological crisis that may impair their ability to make decisions.
         5. Sexual relationships are exploitive because the therapist's power and control in the relationship is always greater than the clients.
22. Your answer should include the idea that the existence and cause of repressed memories is a hotly debated issue. There have been cases where clients and/or family members have successfully brought suit, charging that therapists had intentionally implanted false memories, usually of sexual abuse.
23. a. Your answer should include the idea that managed care systems allocate services in order to contain costs.
     b. They are opposed, because there are incentives to put economic profits before quality of care. Also, clinical judgements regarding the decision of whether or not to provide treatment and the type and level of treatment, is made by a case manager, who is often not a mental health professional.
24. a. The principles endorsed by a profession that encourage and forbid certain types of conduct and express the profession's norms and aspirations.
     b. limiting practice to areas of demonstrated competence, maintaining proper clinical records, using and interpreting tests properly, protecting the privacy and confidentiality of client communications, consulting and cooperating with other mental health professionals, eliminating bias, protecting that client's welfare
25. a. basic scientists--develop basic understanding about issues which may, at some point, relate to the legal system
     b. trial consultants--aid in jury selection and trial preparation
     c. policy evaluators or researchers--study the effects of changes in correctional programs, legislation or social services
     d. expert witnesses--testify in civil and criminal trials
26. a. They are specialty fields which apply mental health knowledge to questions about individuals involved in legal proceedings.
     b. 1. There are many different topics about which mental health experts can testify.
         2. The law permits and even encourages it.
         3. It is possible for forensic experts to earn thousands of dollars per case.
27. In order to be judged as incompetent to stand trial, a defendant must, because of his or her mental disorder: (1) be unable to understand the nature of the trial proceedings, (2) be unable to participate meaningfully in their own defense or (3) be unable to consult with their attorney.

28.

INSANITY STANDARD	DATE	SUMMARY
McNaughton Rule	1843	To be judged NGRI the person must, at the time of the act, either not know what he or she was doing or not understand that his actions were wrong.
Durham Rule	1954	A person is judged NGRI, if the criminal act was due to mental disorder.
ALI Rule	1972	To be judged NGRI the person, at the time of the act, does not have the capacity to appreciate the wrongfulness of the act or the ability to conform to legal requirements.

29. a. False. Across the United States, fewer than 1 percent of all criminal cases involve a finding of NGRI.
b. False. Defendants found NGRI seldom go completely free.
c. True.
d. False. Studies have found no socioeconomic or racial bias in the use or success of the insanity plea.
e. True.

30. Your answers should include the ideas that:
a. the guilty but mentally ill verdict, which is used in about 25 percent of the states, results in a sentence for an equivalent amount of time beginning in a treatment facility and, after competition of treatment, transfer to a prison. The effectiveness of the GBMI verdict is questioned, it is confusing to juries and treatment in overcrowded facilities is often nonexistent.
b. the Insanity Defense Reform Act was designed to limit the number of defendants in federal courts who successfully claim insanity as a defense. The Act: 1) placed the burden of insanity proof on the defendant, 2) did away with the rule that defined insanity as the inability to control conduct and 3) restricted the testimony of expert witnesses to descriptions of mental conditions only, not conclusions.
c. even though a few states have abolished the insanity defense, consideration of the defendant's state of mind at the time of the alleged crime is still important. In order to prove guilt, intent (and therefore competence) must also be proven.